OPEN ALL NIGHT

KEN MILLER

OPEN ALL NIGHT

with text by

WILLIAM T. VOLLMANN

The Overlook Press
Woodstock • New York

FOR
PEARL AND
SALVATORE

First published in 1995 by
The Overlook Press
Lewis Hollow Road
Woodstock, New York 12498

The Rainbow Stories, Thirteen Stories and Thirteen Epigraphs, The Ice-Shirt and Butterfly Stories were first published by André Deutsch Limited. Whores For Gloria was first published by Pan Books Ltd, London. The short story "Red and Blue" first appeared in SPIN Magazine.

Library of Congress Cataloging-in-Publication Data
Miller, Ken
Open all night / Ken Miller; text by William T. Vollmann. p. cm.
1. Portrait photography. 2. Punk culture—United States—Pictorial works. 3. Psychiatric hospital patients—United States—Portraits. 4. Narcotic addicts—United States—Portraits. 5. Prostitutes—United States—Portraits. 6. Miller, Ken, 1963-
I. Vollmann, William T. II. Title.
TR680.M48 1995
779'.930568—dc20 95-17594 CIP

Printed and bound at Meridian Printing, East Greenwich, Rhode Island
Photograph negatives by Thomas Palmer
Book design by Michael Hornburg
Typeset by AeroType, Inc.

ISBN: 0-87951-648-8 (PB)
ISBN: 0-87951-571-6 (HC)
First Edition

ACKNOWLEDGMENTS

There have been many people who have helped in the production of this book and I would like to extend my thanks first to Mr. Jock Sturges, who has been a teacher and friend for over a decade. Jock's kind support of cameras, lenses, film, paper, a darkroom, a floor to sleep on, and a hot meal was very much appreciated during the many years I lived on the streets. I would also like to thank Mr. William T. Vollmann, a true friend and the most dangerous man I have ever met. Bill's words have carried my photographs to many places. His generous gifts of trips to Burma, Thailand and Cambodia have helped to enrich my life and my work like nothing else. Further thanks go out to my father, who first taught me how to use a camera; my mother, who let me use the camera; my grandparents and Sally and Vups, my first models; Mr. Walter Goodrich, who taught me about people; Mr. Tsang, my first photography teacher, who taught me the power of the camera; Mr. Harvey Levine, who taught me how to see without using a camera; Mr. Mark McMaster; Mr. Dave Soter, Mr. Paul Girard and Mr. Ben Pax for bringing me to California; Mr. John Gangidino and the many other sheet rockers and tapers who employed me; Mr. Harrison J. Sheppard, my attorney and friend, whose brilliance and encouragement keeps me in perspective; my cousin Lee Miller for printing the pictures in this book; Mr. Davis Pratt; Mr. & Mrs. James Lombino; Ms. Florence Jesmajian; Mr. Spencer Weisbroth; Mr. Steven Goldstine; Mr. Joe Foelberg; Mr. Joel Leivick; Ms. Laura Volkerding; Mr. Paul Kos; Ms. Marlene Zullo, Ms. Jen Kos; Mr. Steven Shapiro; Mr. Simon Lowinsky; Mr. Tom Myer; the Brock Family; Ms. Caroline Cabading; Mr. Richard Marcel; Mr. Walter Sunday; The San Francisco Art Institute; The Maine Photographer's Workshops; Stanford University; The 509 Cultural Center/Luggage Store Annex; Vision Gallery; Lowinsky Gallery; The 441 Club. Above all, I would like to thank Marisa and Brittania, Lee, Cammie Toloui-Kotchetkov, Howard, The Kickboxing Association of Thailand, Shizue, the street alcoholics of Haight Street, the San Francisco Neo Nazi Skinheads, and all the pimps, whores, and drug dealers of the Tenderloin. God Bless.

OPEN AL

I sometimes think that Ken Miller would prefer to treat the world with the honeyed blandness of a high-priced psychiatrist, accepting of all, pleasantly inscrutable, wise and tired. He avoids defining his photographic project; he avoids it in an insistent, aggressive, irritating way. If pressed to explain what he is doing, he will, if he is feeling extremely good-humored, put on a smile of what must be deliberately crafted stupidity, and say something like, "I'm taking these pictures just to document." Yet the truth is that Ken is no camera eye, tumbling in magisterial orbit from pole to pole, clicking every three point four seconds on whatever has shown itself to be documented in that interval; for he has strong dislikes. What most people call beauty annoys him; what they call riches disgusts him, and the manners of his own class, the middle class, incite him to grinning personal taunts. This genuinely ugly side of his character frames his work, because it is what is called the *ugly* that attracts him. He will forgive you your theories if you limp or have a cast in one eye. A thug hideously tattooed, a street witch whose rat-familiar peers out from between her breasts, a stinking bum who pisses in Ken's sink—these are the people who will open the shutters of his heart to maximum aperture, like a high school girl who was just given a rose. But it is not that he is a mere pornographer of the abnormal. There are too many of those; we see their productions every week in the magazines—sometimes a starving African child with a bloated belly, and other times the clutching fingers of a dying earthquake victim. These images soothe people's passivity because they do not teach them anything. What makes Ken's work so remarkable is the sense that these squashed lives are not just isolated bugs on the windshield, but *parallel worlds* of hermetic secrets, like the nine cities of Troy stacked one upon the next inside the earth. This comes across in part because Ken takes many different pictures of his subjects at different times and places, but he is able to do that only because he knows his subjects and gets them to trust him. You can see it in the way they look at the camera. Imagine the excitement of the fellow who discovered Pluto through his calculations, realizing gradually from the color temperature of his integrals that there was something cold and black and unknown far out there, following our sun its own way, and it had been there forever but we had never known that it was there. That was how I felt one afternoon when Ken took me to Golden Gate Park, five minutes away from the playground, five minutes away from the bus stop, into a little

L N I G H T

thicket of wet stinking trees, and he introduced me to the Wrecking Crew on their mattresses, with their sad alcoholic lore about Smackwater Jack and the wild blue yonder. It was not that he had shown me a group of tramps who had been living in the Park for years that impressed me. It was that he knew them by name and they knew him, and that was the open sesame for me to understand that they had an identity and a place; that this was their kingdom with its own rules and stories and lice; and that in fact the whole world was like that, and if somebody had enough time he could map it out into these kingdoms (how many millions of them must there be in San Francisco alone?) and *document* them, as Ken would say, before they burst like rainbow-colored soap bubbles. Thanks to Ken I was able to meet the S.F. Skinz in the turning year of their decline, to meet the secret clan of old electroshock patients who lived in fly-infested hotels whose floors were rubbery with their puke, to draw in rough outlines the world-frame of the streetwalkers and the trainhoppers, and, most importantly, to understand that every person is like an exotic book, and if you go to the trouble of reading it you will learn about things that you had never imagined. I hope that someday Ken will crack the private worlds of the secretaries and the grocery store proprietors. I do not think that would weaken his focus. It would be wonderful if he did begin to *document* everybody. But at the moment his interest is in "lost souls" (his words). It is a fine sight to see him walking down the streets with his heavy view camera slung over his shoulder, and his watchdog padding alongside, ready to bite any enemy. He has a very young face, and bright eyes. He wears a faded denim jacket. His hands are calloused and cracked. Every few steps, he will see somebody that he recognizes. He stops, yells: "Hey, Smiley! *Kirby!* How ya doin'? *Laddie!* When did you get into town?" He has pictures for all of them. They come running, hopping or hobbling. They love him because he gives them pictures. When the clutch the new images in their hands, so happy and proud, anyone can see that they are not as lost as you or I might think, or want to think. And if they are lost, it may be because they want to be one of those undiscovered black planets spinning so quietly and secretly that most people never find it, never meet its kings and warriors, never run their fingers through its cold black treasure.

– William T. Vollmann

OPEN ALL NIGHT

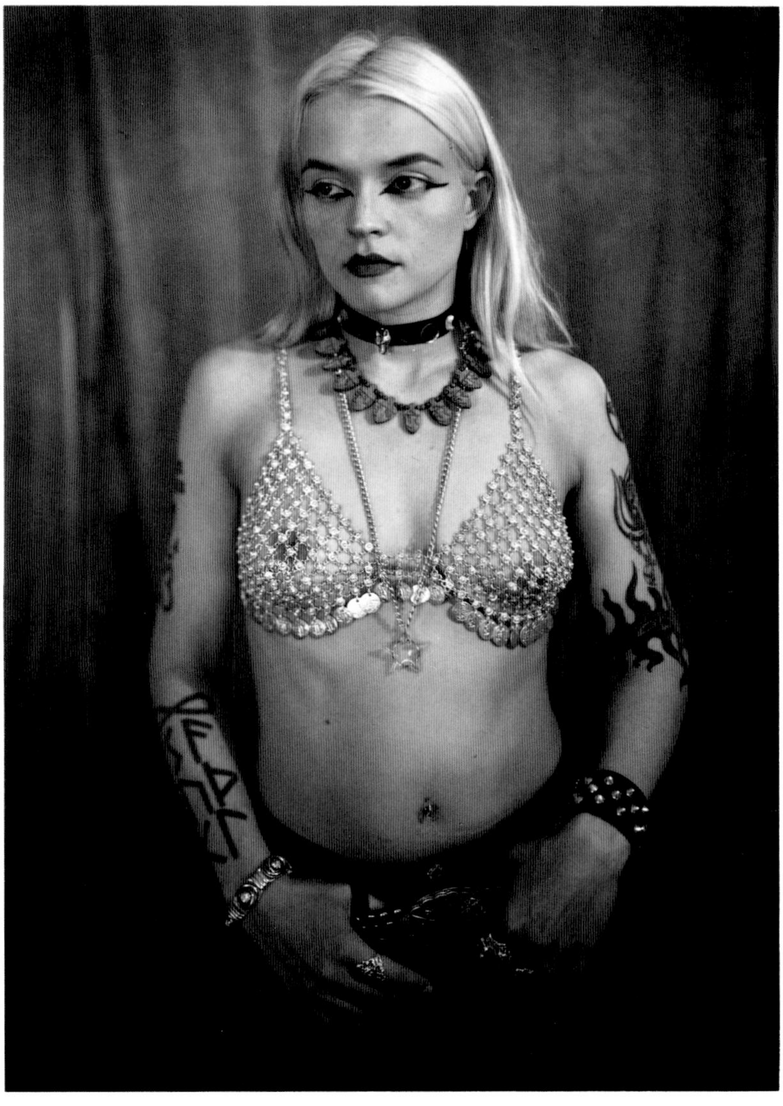

. . . so once upon a time Ken happened to be driving slowly down a Tenderloin street looking for Brownie, his favorite black girlfriend who wanted to be his girlfriend and had even offered to fuck him in the North Star Laundromat, but on this most momentous afternoon Ken saw, instead of Brownie, a young Japanese woman standing very mournfully on the corner and I wish I could describe the beauty of her smooth face whose eyes conveyed nothing and her black glory of hair, which fell down to her breasts as she leaned a little forward with her lips pursed, looking at Ken in a way that he had never seen before . . .

"The Ghost of Magnetism"
THIRTEEN STORIES AND THIRTEEN EPIGRAPHS

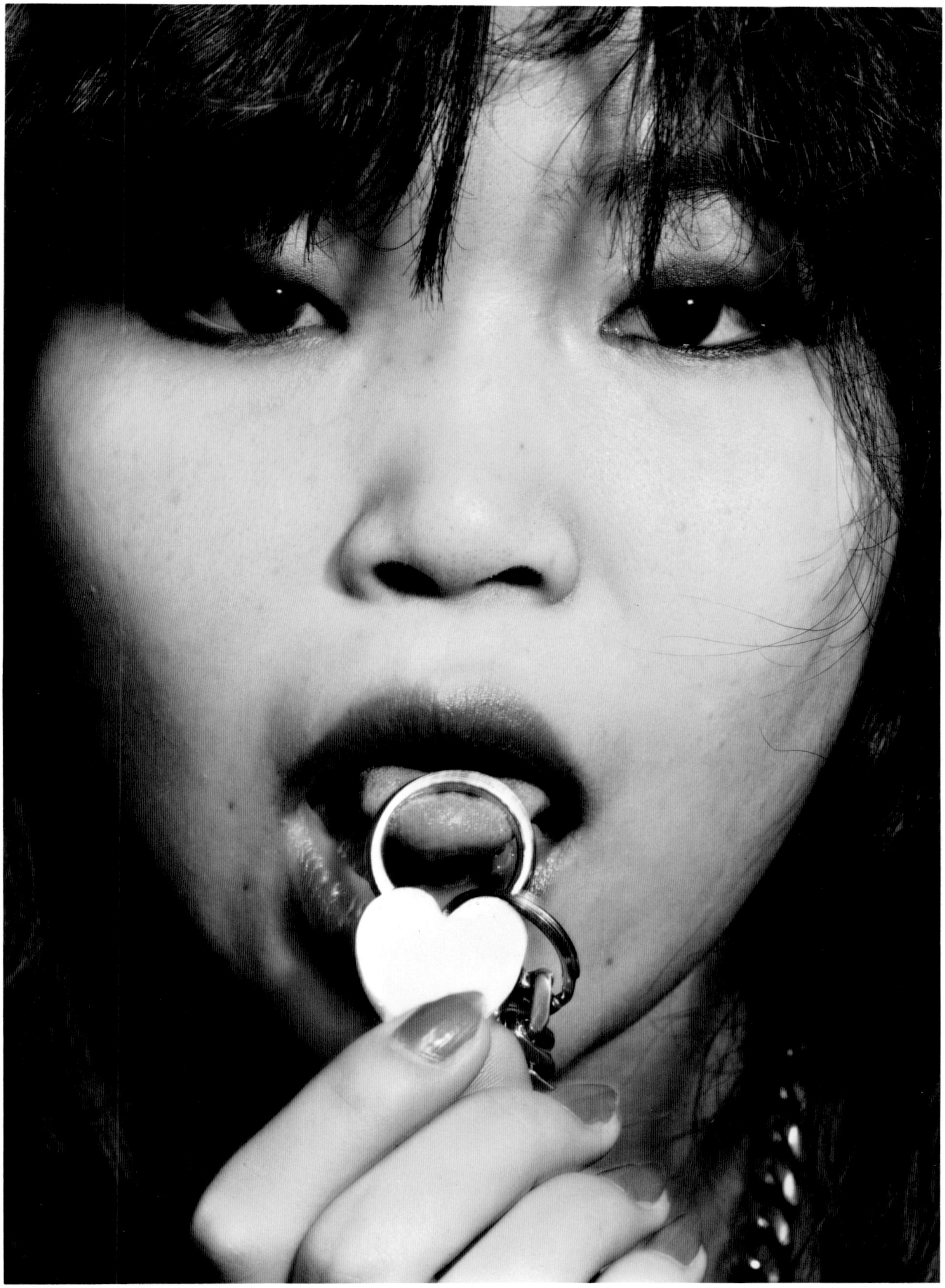

See, there's this *awesome* park that Elaine can take you to, said Carmella. They've got steel trees and steel benches and when you put a quarter in these steel benches come and fold over your lap so you're protected.

"The Handcuff Manual"
THIRTEEN STORIES AND THIRTEEN EPIGRAPHS

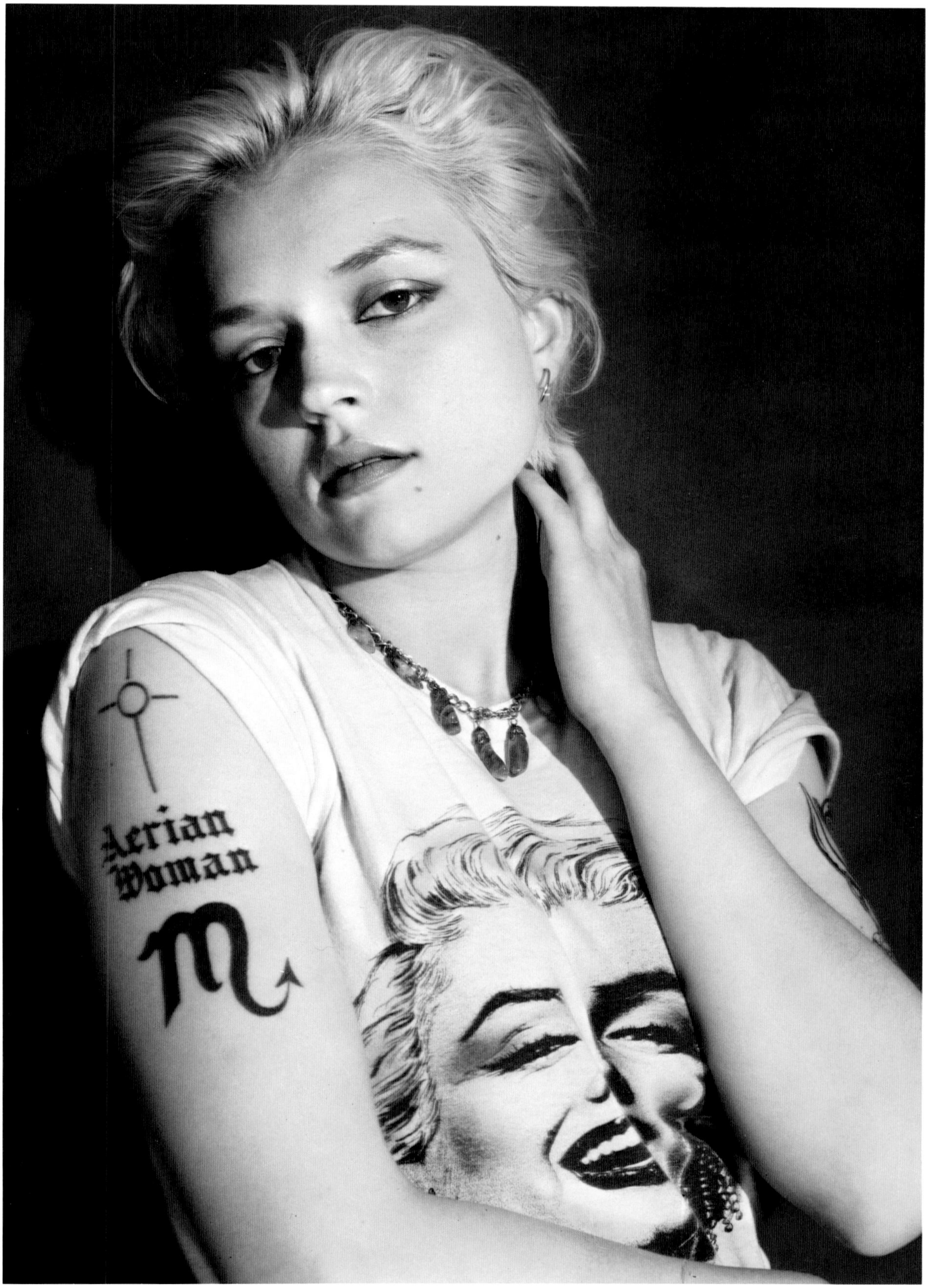
Aerian
Woman

You trying to apologize for something? You think you got something to apologize for? I got more to apologize for than you ever dreamed. You try and pull a fast one and apologize first. I say no way, Jose. I say you better listen, cocksucker.

"Flowers in Your Hair"
THIRTEEN STORIES AND THIRTEEN EPIGRAPHS

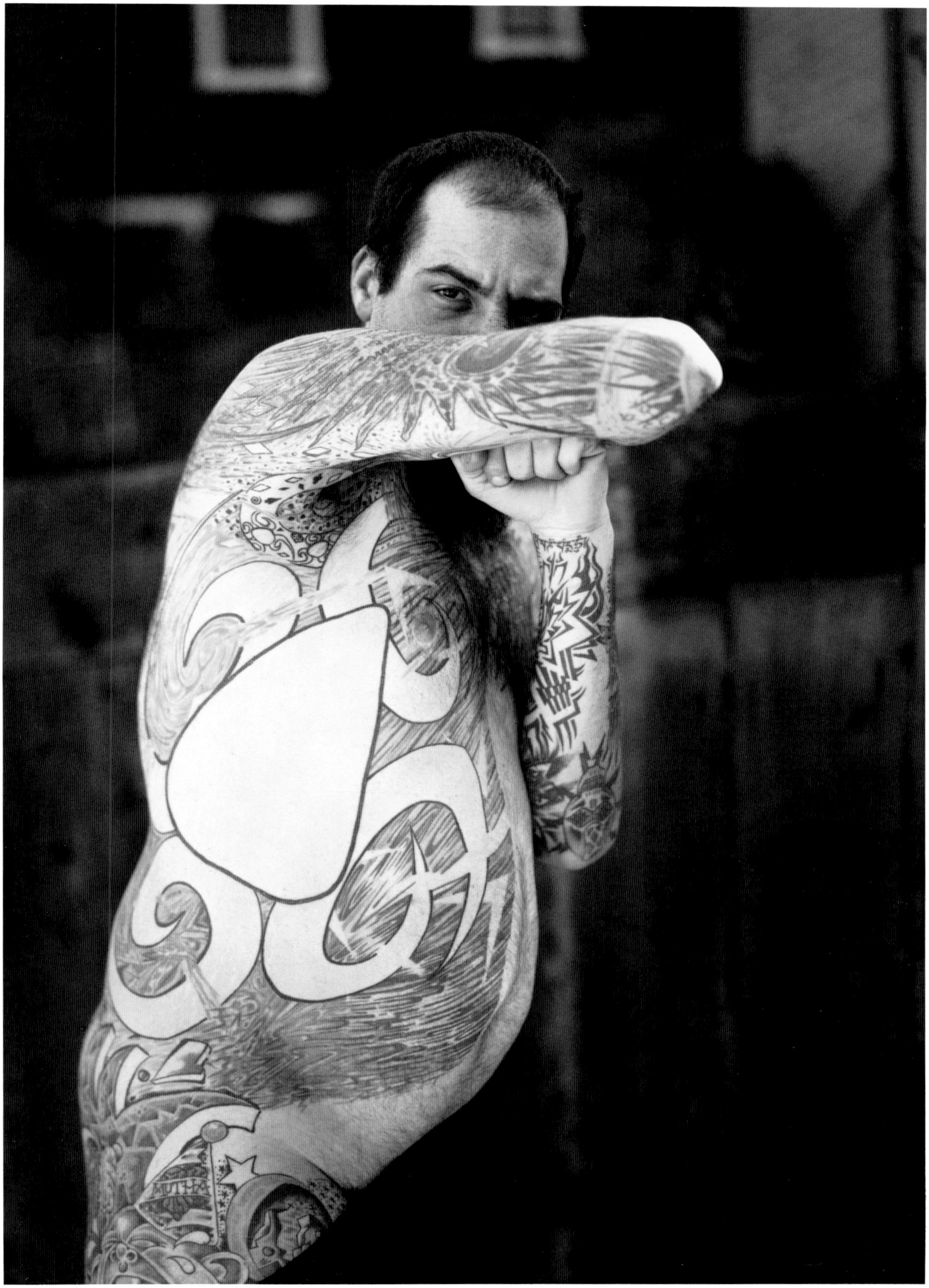

"You weren't supposed to make me feel desperate, because you weren't supposed to love me," said the TV.

"Violet Hair"
THE RAINBOW STORIES

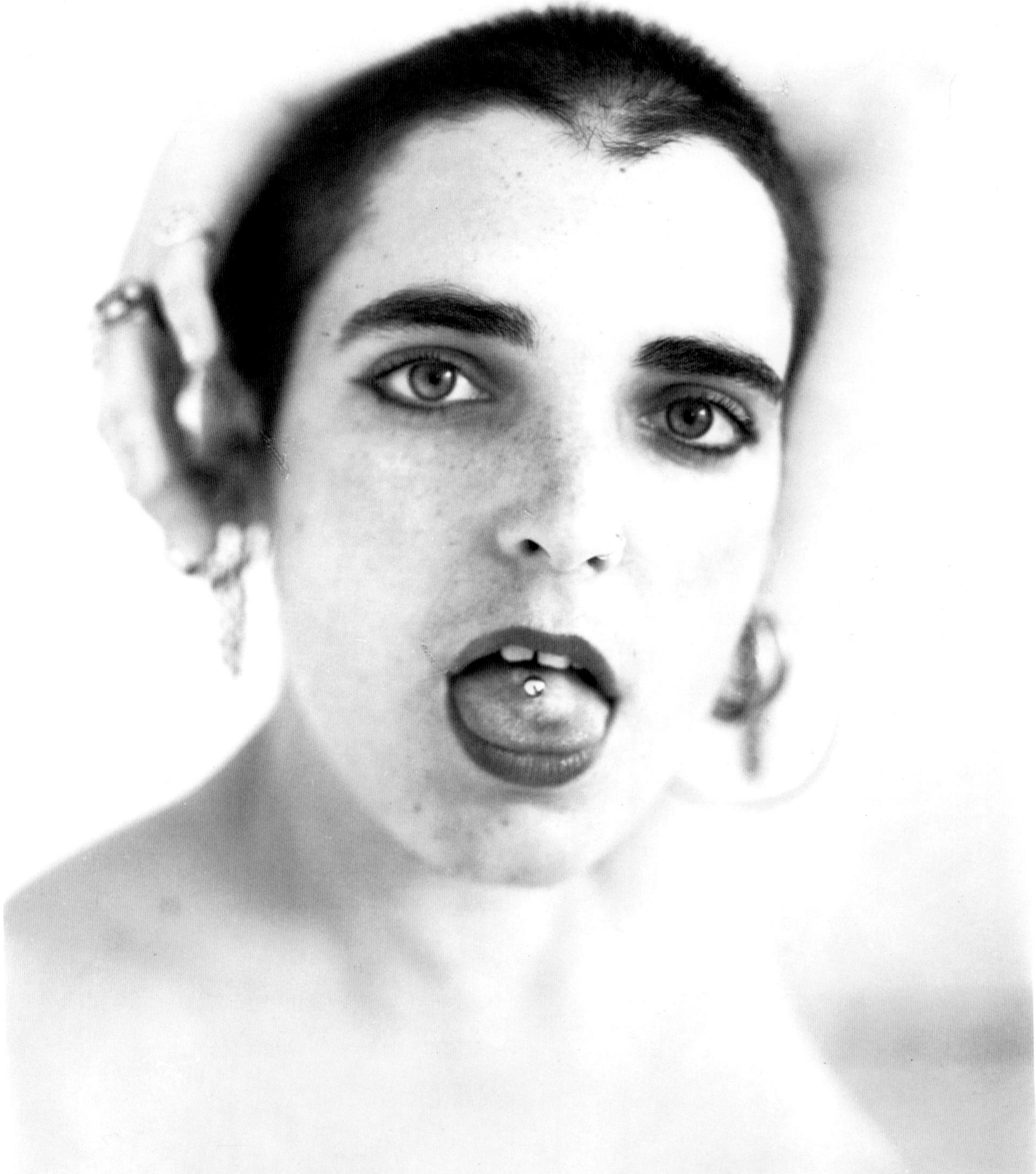

They came in already half loaded, and Joy had bought a giant-sized Singha beer for each of them. Pukki sat on the journalist's bed scarcely paying any attention to him; her face was full of Joy, who lay hugging the photographer and glancing over her shoulder every ten minutes or so at Pukki, who would giggle again; the photographer had said he thought they were lesbians which the journalist hadn't believed, but now he wondered and said quietly to Pukki: You go with ladies sometimes? and Pukki blushed and said: Sometimes and he said: You go with Joy sometimes? and she nodded. —He said to her: You no want stay with me? It's OK, honey. I pay you same you stay, same you no stay; up to you . . . —and Pukki whirled on him in a flash, scared now, and started snuggling him, and he felt very sad. —I stay I stay! she whispered. I stay short-time you want short-time; I stay all night you want all night! and this got his hopes up a little bit; so maybe he'd finally found a Thai lady who'd stay all night with him (all the photographer's had been all-nights), so he said: OK, you stay all night, please, Pukki and she smiled. —Joy said something to her very sharply and she opened her fingers to show him a condom and said: You use this please. —That's only fair, he said. I've been telling you I'm a butterfly. —Butterfly no problem me, she said.

Butterfly Stories

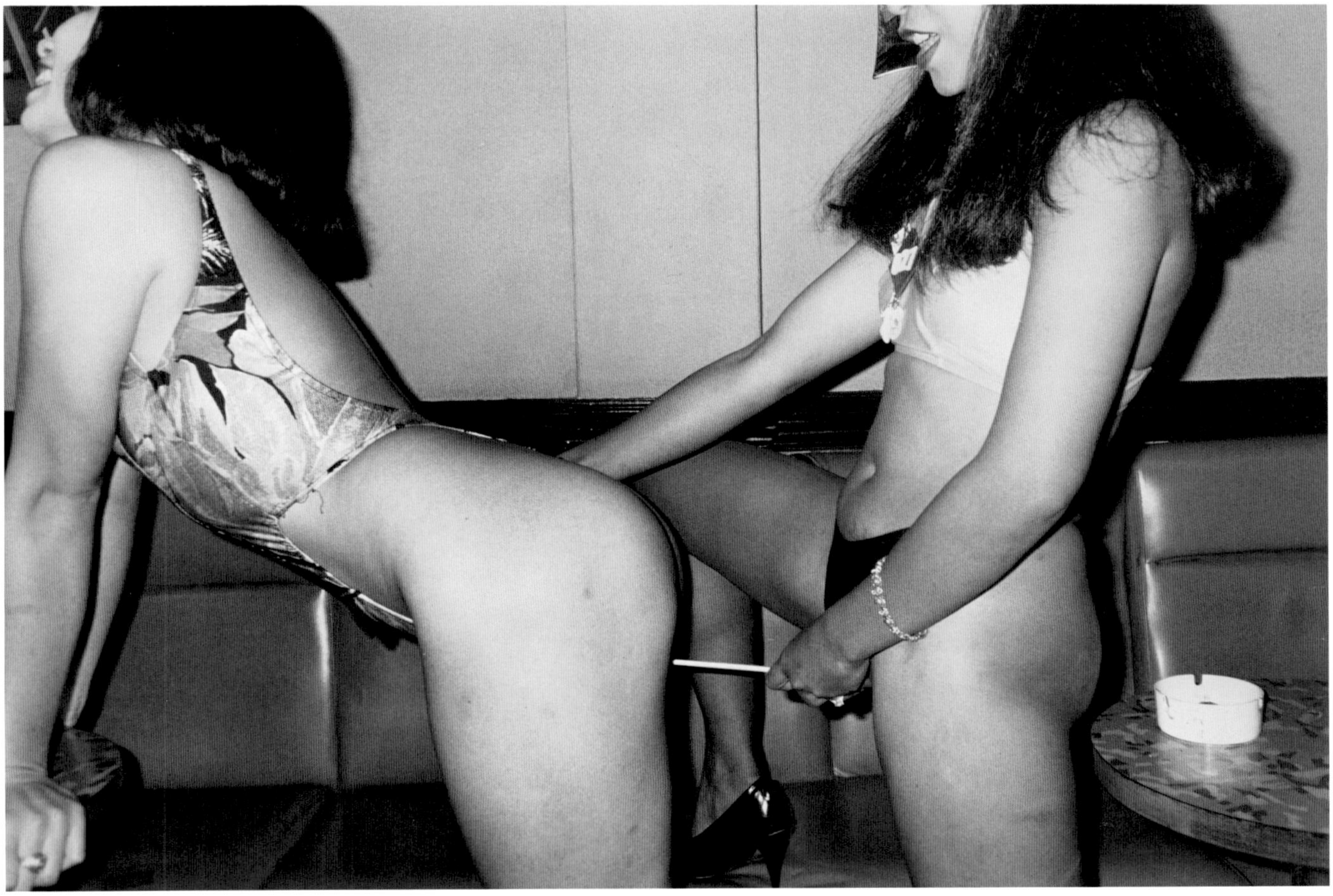

Red shot a leg up to get Blue in the stomach. Blue did not flinch. Both kept their gloves above their faces. Red got an arm around Blue's neck. Blue punched him behind, hissing *isss!* and threw Blue down. Arising less than easily. Blue gripped Red in an expressionless embrace which somehow involved the side of a foot against a knee. This was life, was life's bitter sweat in the hourlong moments between intermissions when silver strings of water drip down the boxer's hair, the centurylong moments when knee meets knee and thigh meets stomach, when the heel finally scores the solar plexus. A leg shot up. Blue's wrist went under Red's knee and threw him. The crowd cried: *Eh! Eh! Eh!*—because that was rare; from few of these moments could anything could be squeezed but continued clinging and struggling. Blue and Red were embracing at the neck, working their knees around each other's legs and buttocks. A glove in the side, but it was always an embrace. They locked knees around each other. More than anything else I'd ever seen, it was like some new and terrible way of making love.

"Red and Blue"
THE ATLAS

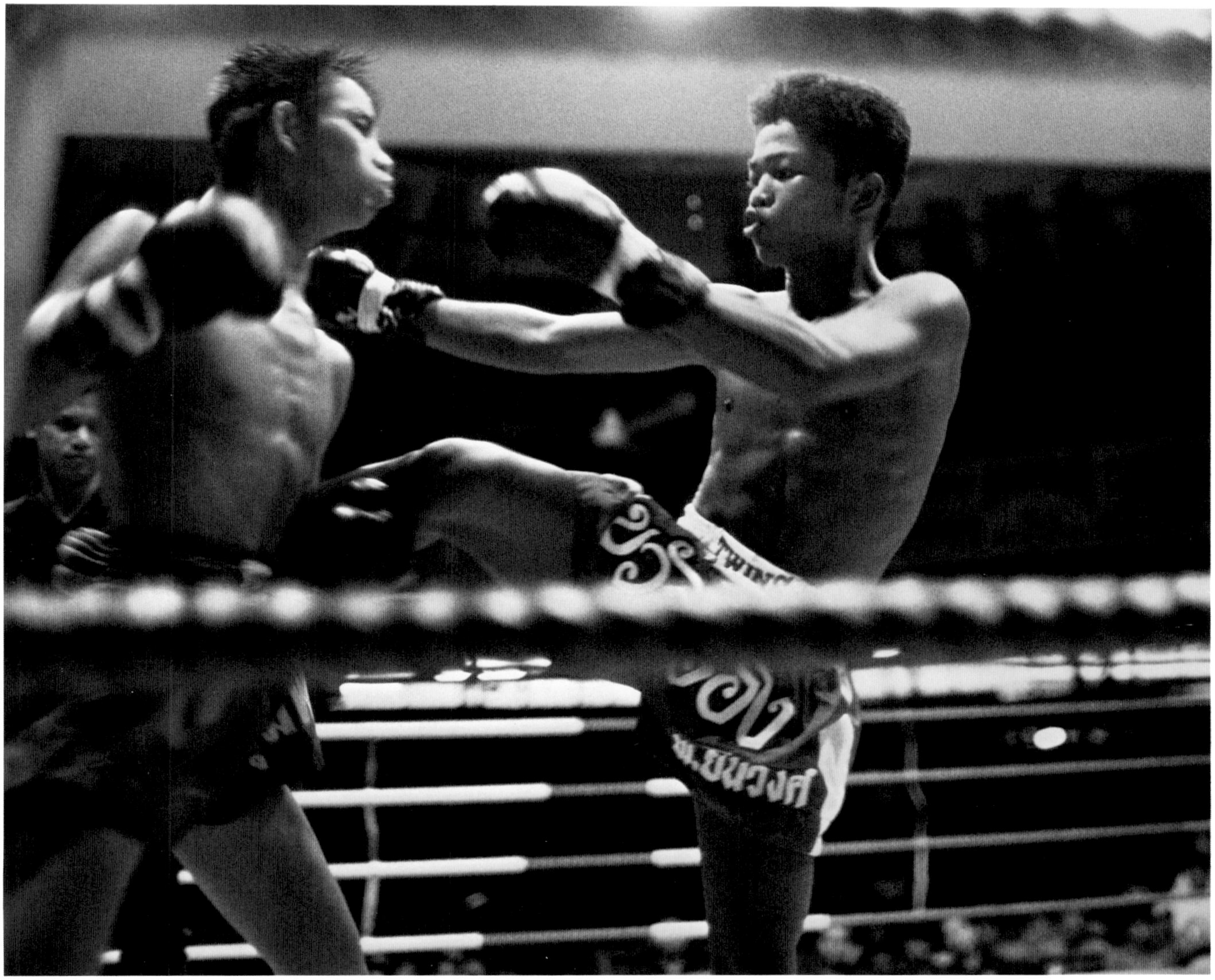

"Politics," I once heard a conservative say, "is the exercise of power. Power is the ability to inflict pain." By this criterion the skinheads are among our most spontaneous politicians. Let us assume, then, that being spontaneous they are light of heart.

"The White Knights"
THE RAINBOW STORIES

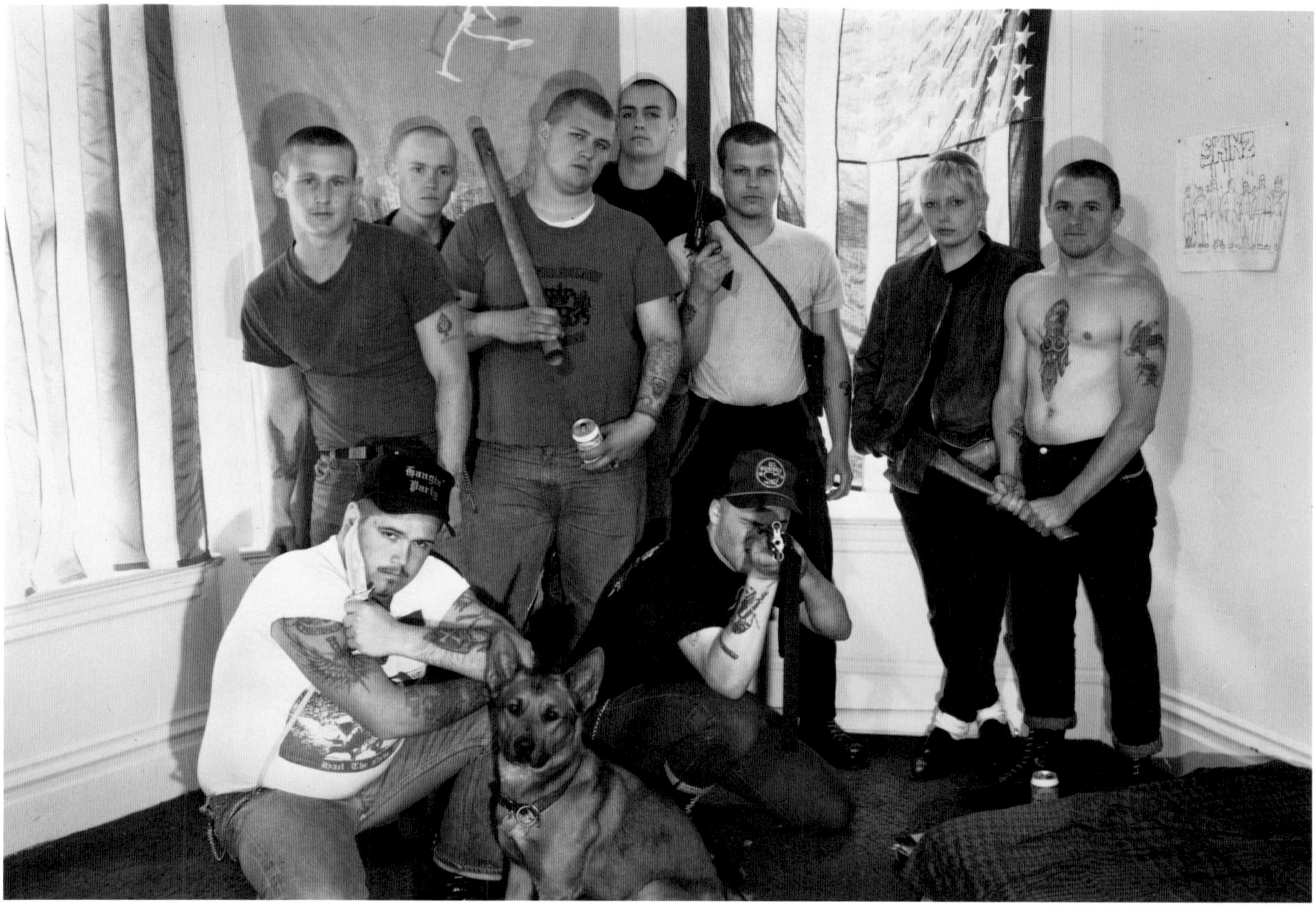
SKINZ
Hangin' Party

They used to go into bars and pick fights, punch people in the face when they didn't like the way they looked (being Nazis, they were conscious that appearance is everything). At least that is what some people said about them. But the Skinz said they didn't start anything. It was the others who started things, who talked rude to them and then didn't get out of the way.

"The White Knights"
THE RAINBOW STORIES

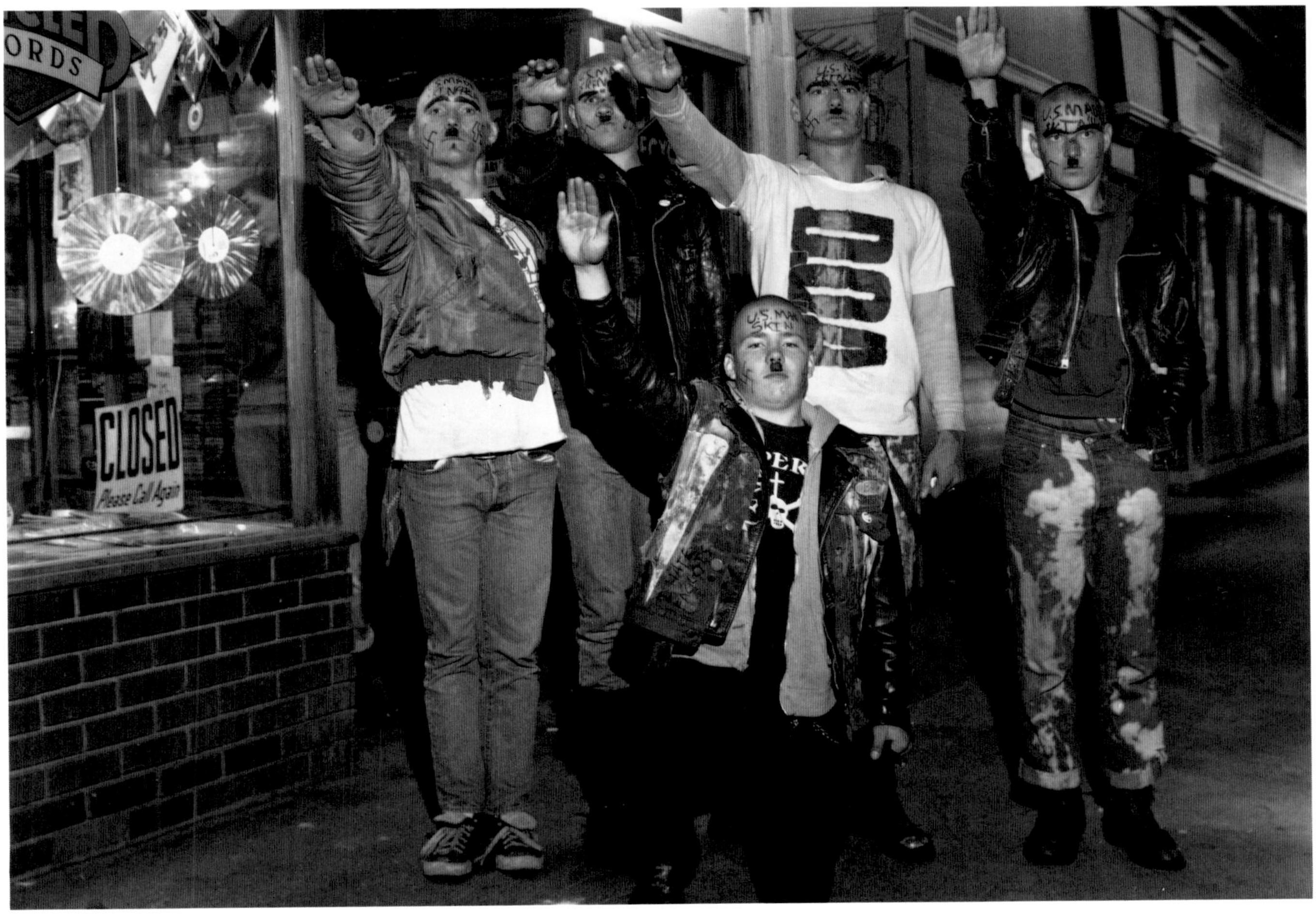
CLOSED
Please Call Again

In a skinhead face, as I have said, eyes become of prime importance.

"The White Knights"
THE RAINBOW STORIES

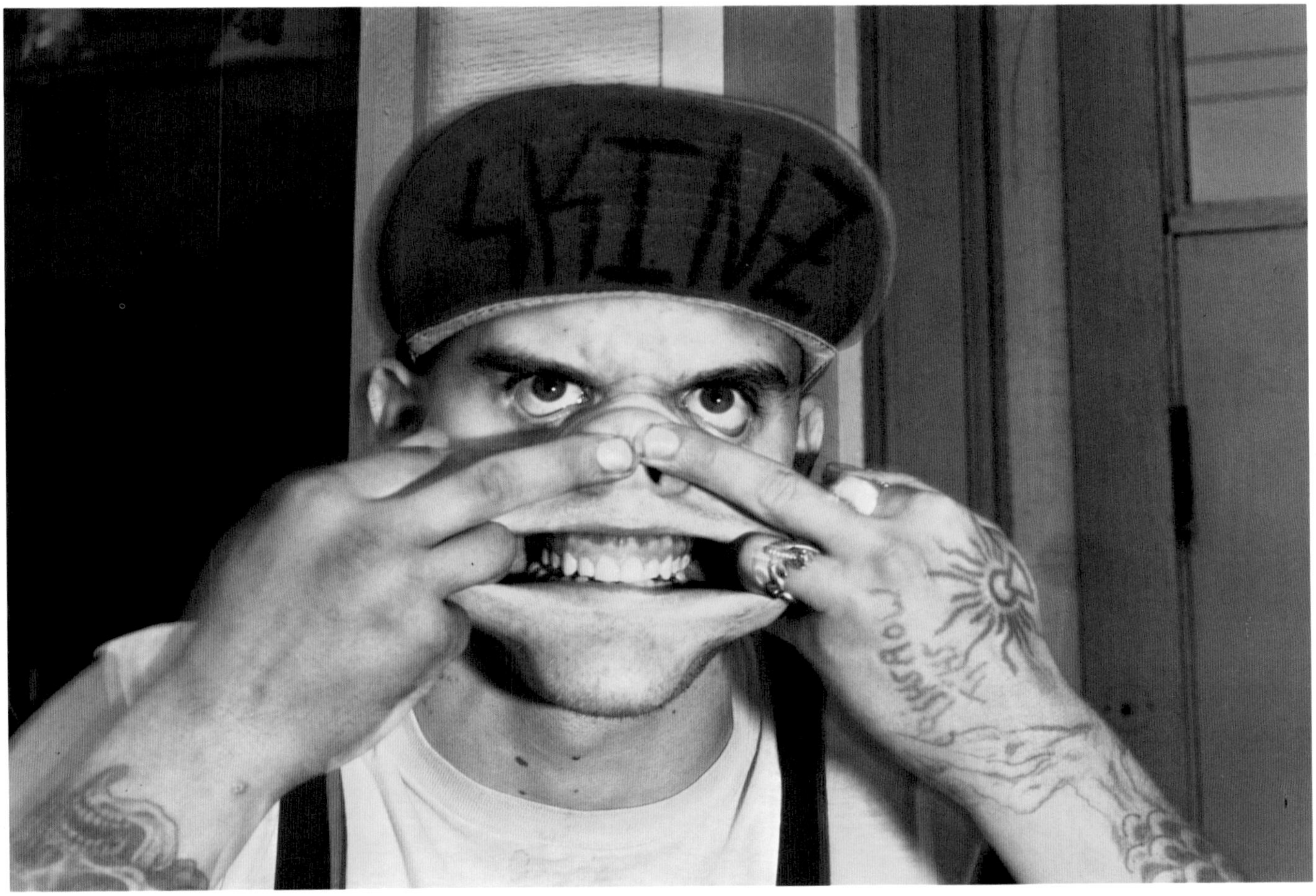
SKINZ

Their shaven heads made them seem particularly thoughtful, with all the profundity of skulls.

"The White Knights"
THE RAINBOW STORIES

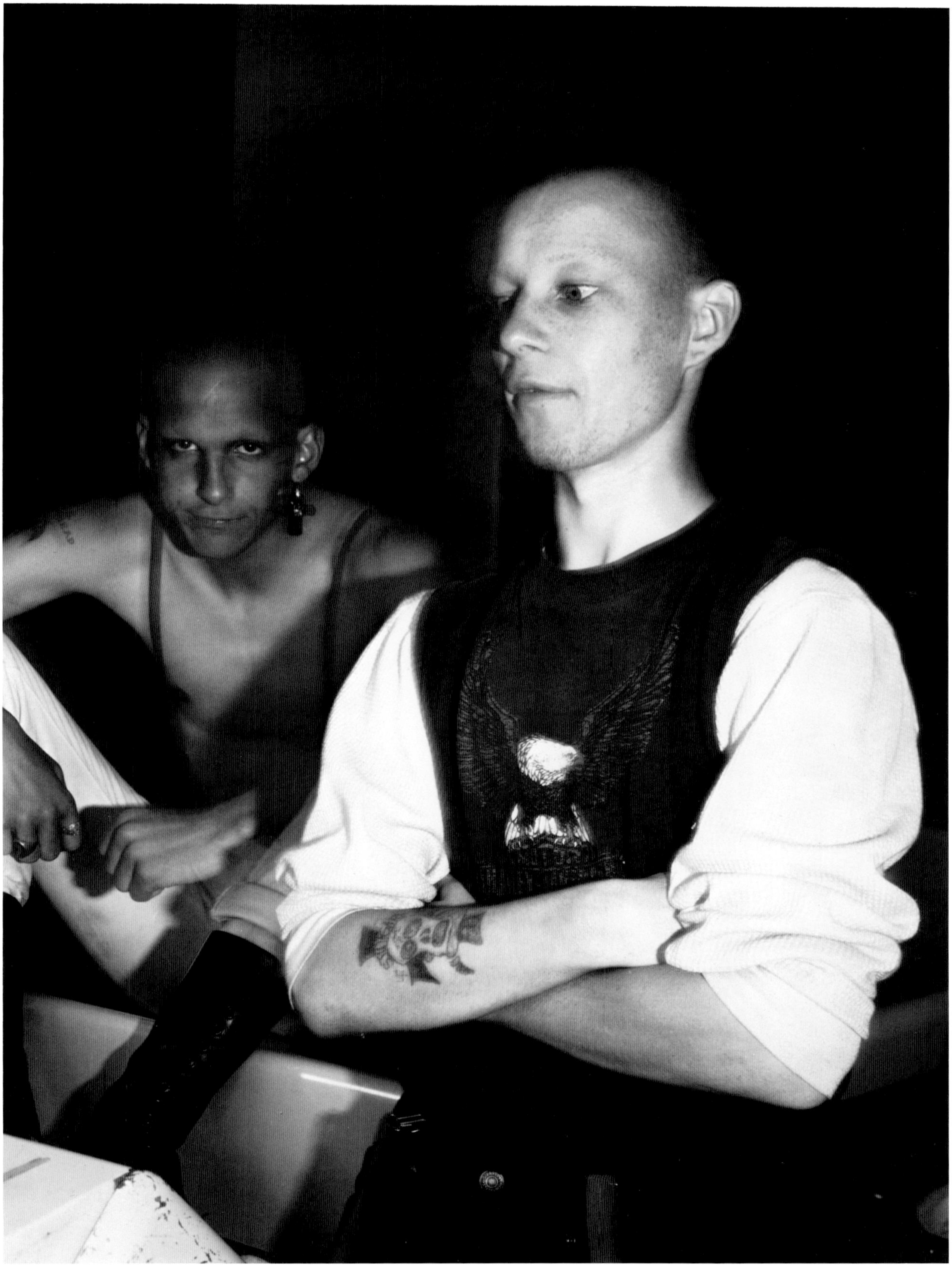

SO BEWARE ENEMYS [sic] OF THE FLAG

"The White Knights"
THE RAINBOW STORIES

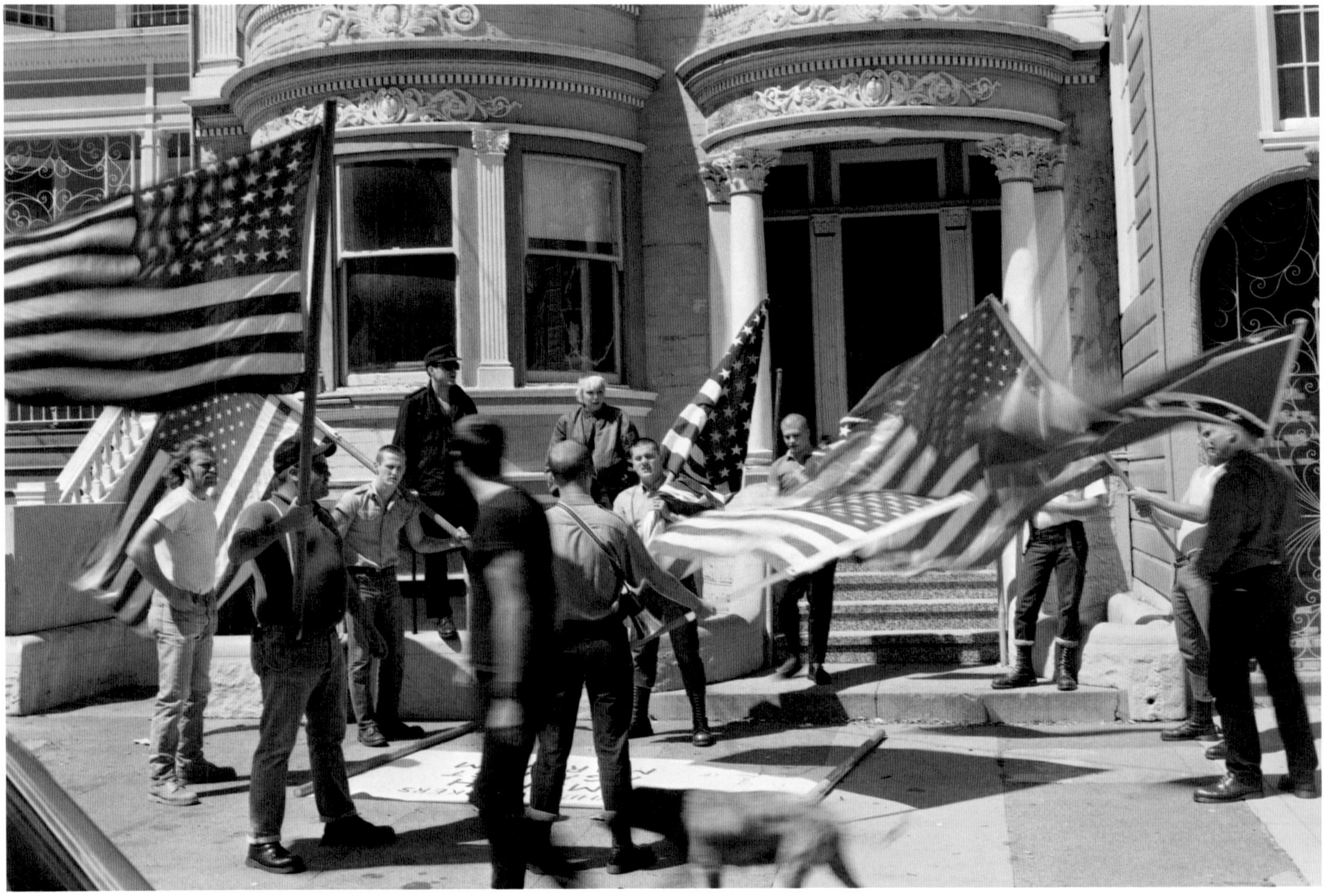

Dickie sat crooning inwardly to the cassette player with his eyes closed, the clean shadow of his head and neck doubling in outline a soldier's helmet upon the kitchen door. Other shadows connected him to the tape player, the two round eyes of its speakers rolling dolefully, like those of an old dog; and Dickie tilted his head back farther, rigidifying the black helmet that he dreamed so freely in; and the shadow of his sleeve flared in one of those venomous elbow-spines sported by insects; and it was impossible to understand what he was thinking; his soul rested in a lone grave beneath the leafless tree of some Civil War battlefield, or wandered through the dugouts of Verdun, steeping from timber to slimy timber with the smell of mud all around him . . .

"The White Knights"
THE RAINBOW STORIES

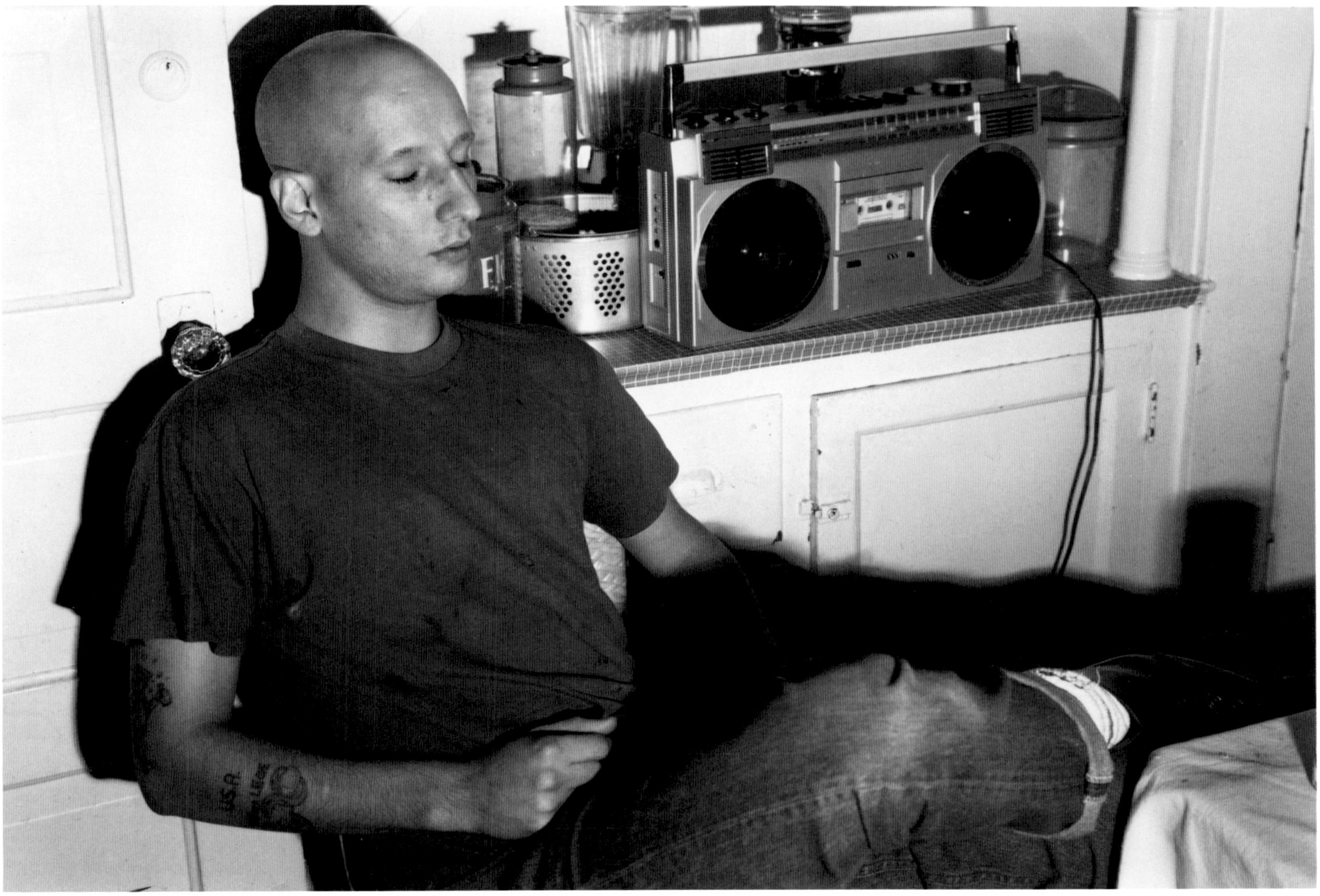

The skinheads lounged in the painted alleys yelling, showing themselves to all as demonic concentration camp traitors.

"The White Knights"
THE RAINBOW STORIES

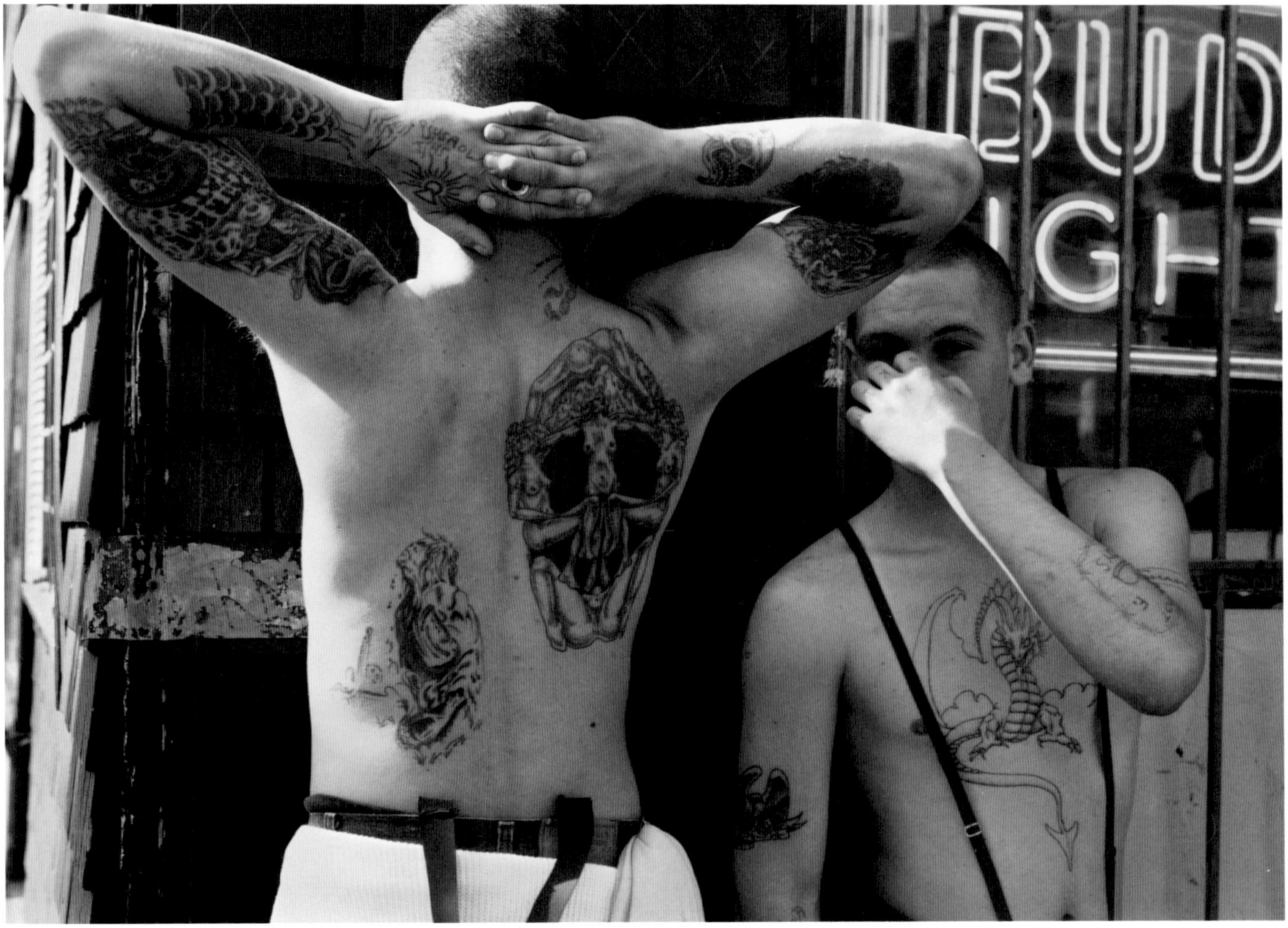
BUD
IGHT

. . . and they said is this a new species or a whole new *genus?*

"The Ghost of Magnetism"
THIRTEEN STORIES AND THIRTEEN EPIGRAPHS

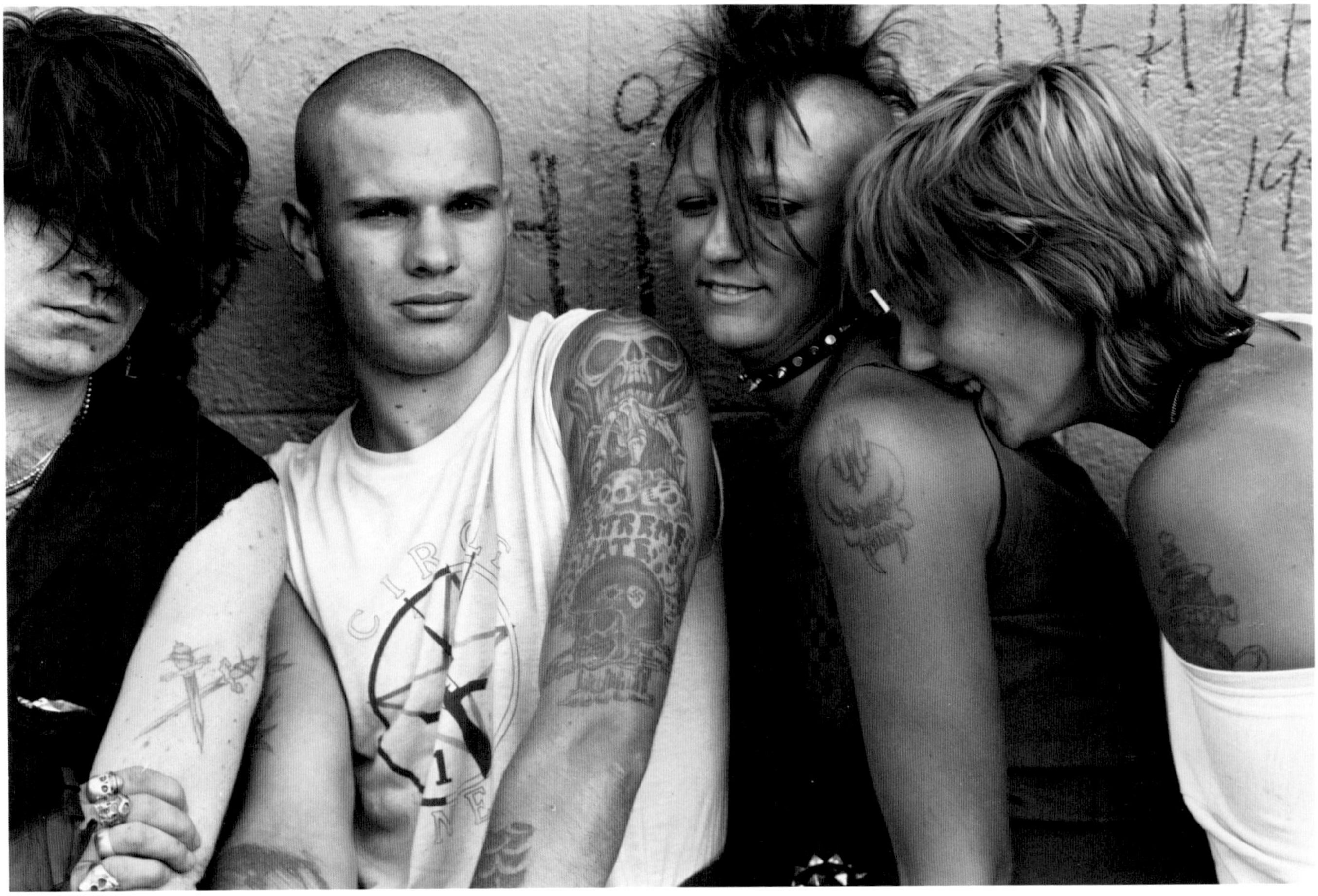

"You gonna beat up the kid?"

"Hell, no," said Dagger, "he's a *skinhead* kid. Someday he'll grow up and make a fine skinhead, a leader, maybe. The person to do that is someone who's raised up on it and knows our law by heart. We started it. It's up to our kids to keep it on."

"The White Knights"
THE RAINBOW STORIES

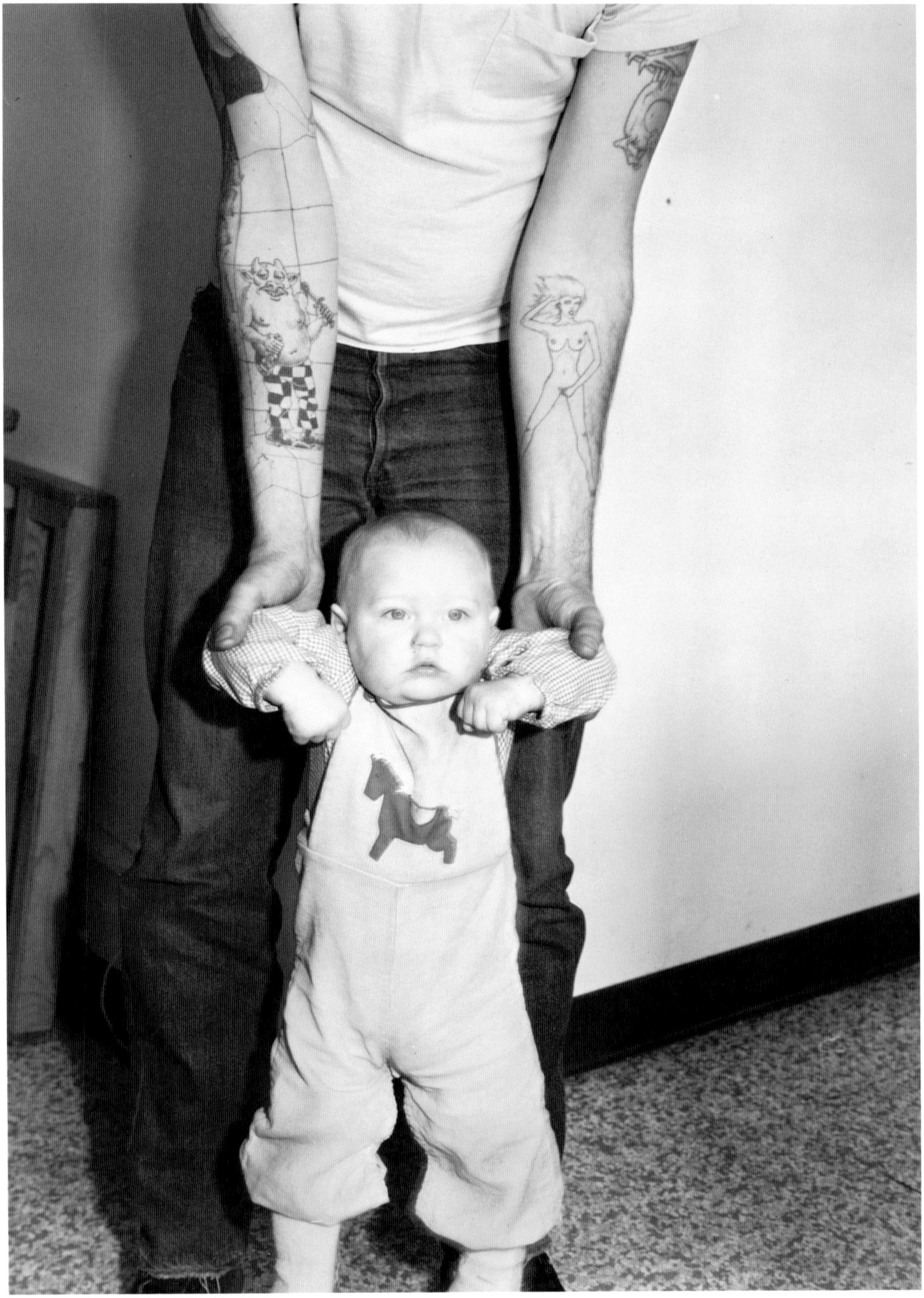

Trustingly she pulled down her pants to show off Bronson's new work on her tattoo whenever I asked. She was my friend.

"The White Knights"
THE RAINBOW STORIES

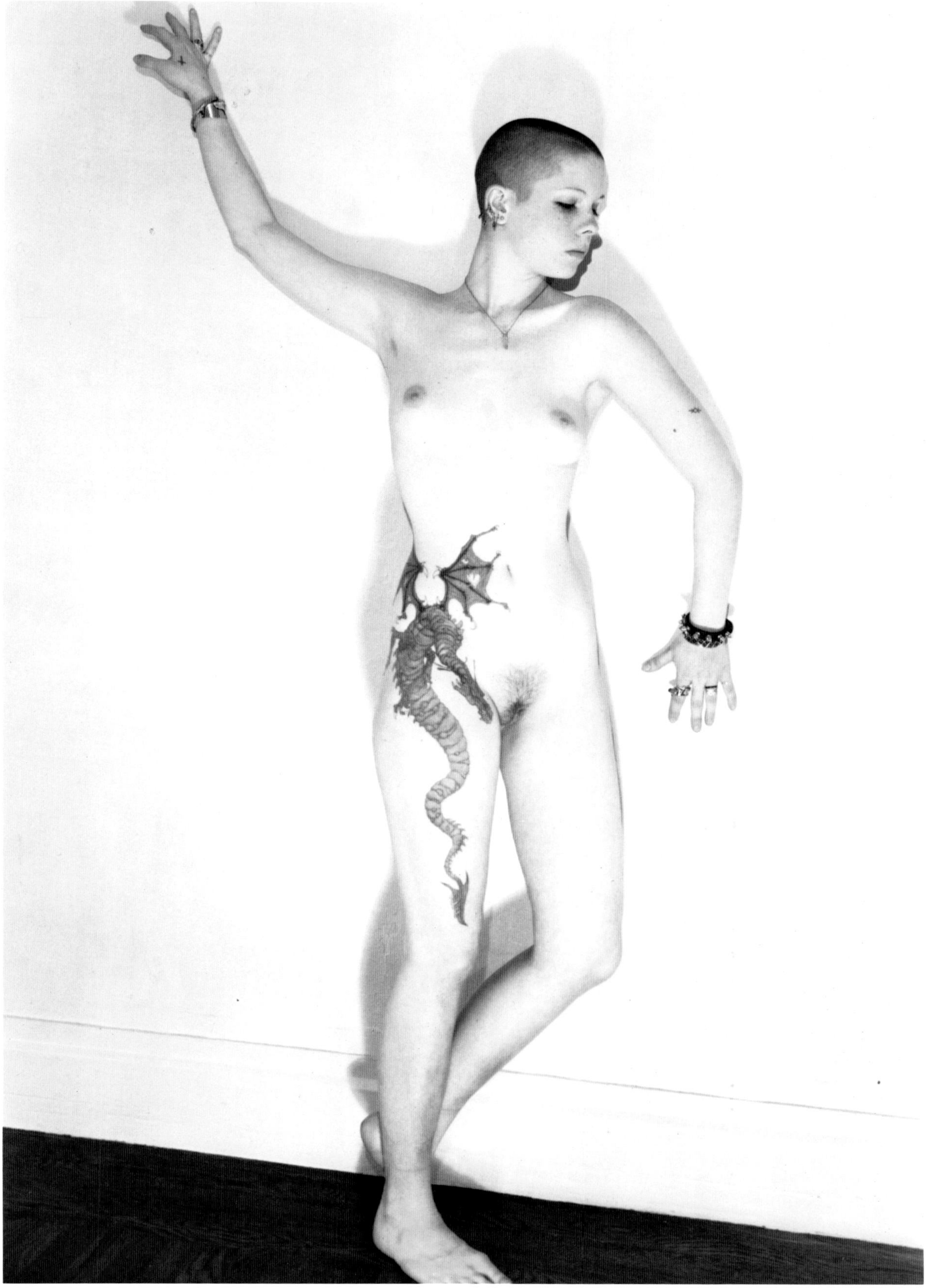

"Almost *all* the skinheads are already dead," sighed Marisa, "all the good ones."

"The Blue Wallet"
THE RAINBOW STORIES

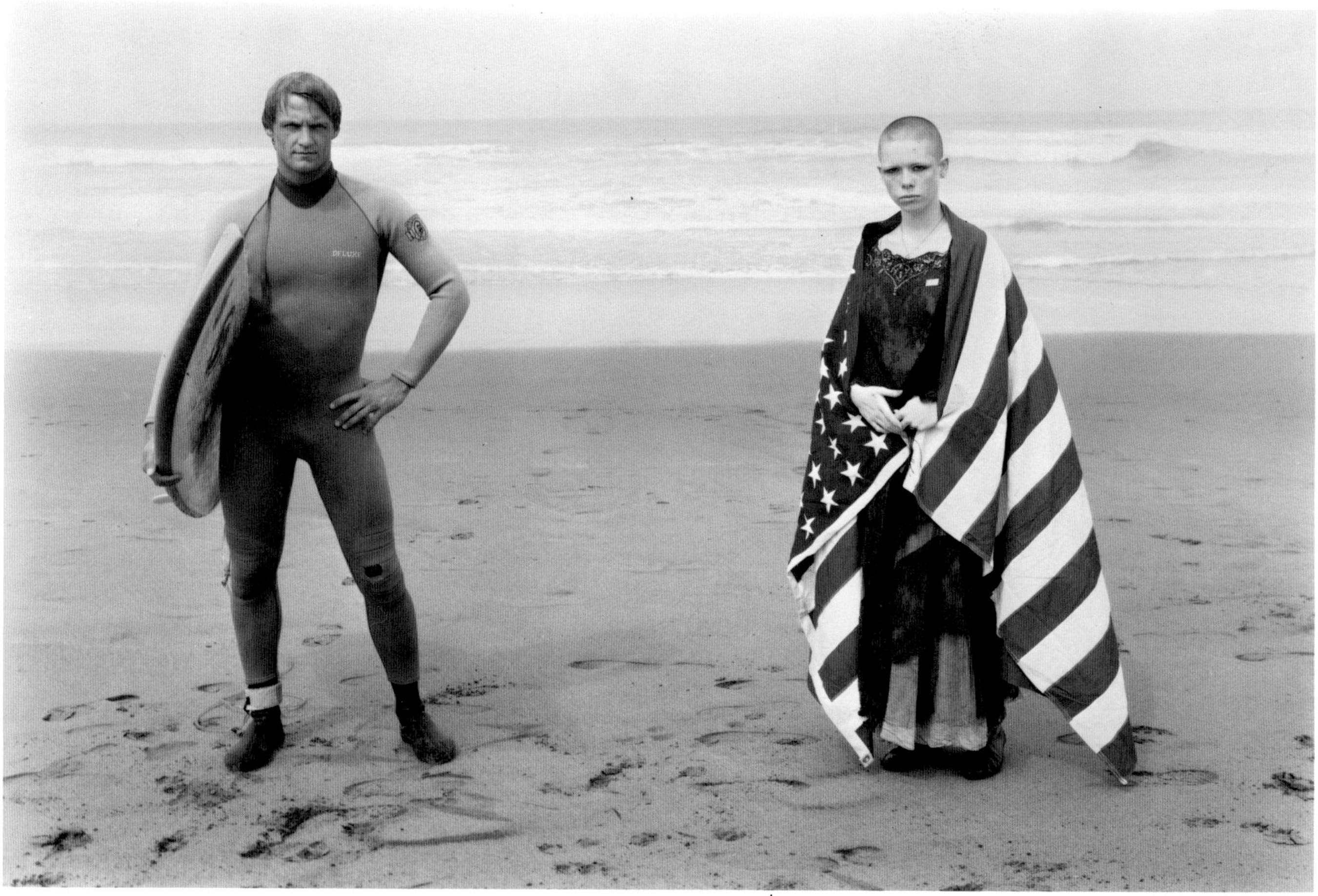

. . . she loved and admired Skinhead Sean, so she tattooed Sean's name on her body and started unrolling her secret capabilities by piercing her ears half a dozen times and doing fucked-up things to her hair.

"The Blue Wallet"
THE RAINBOW STORIES

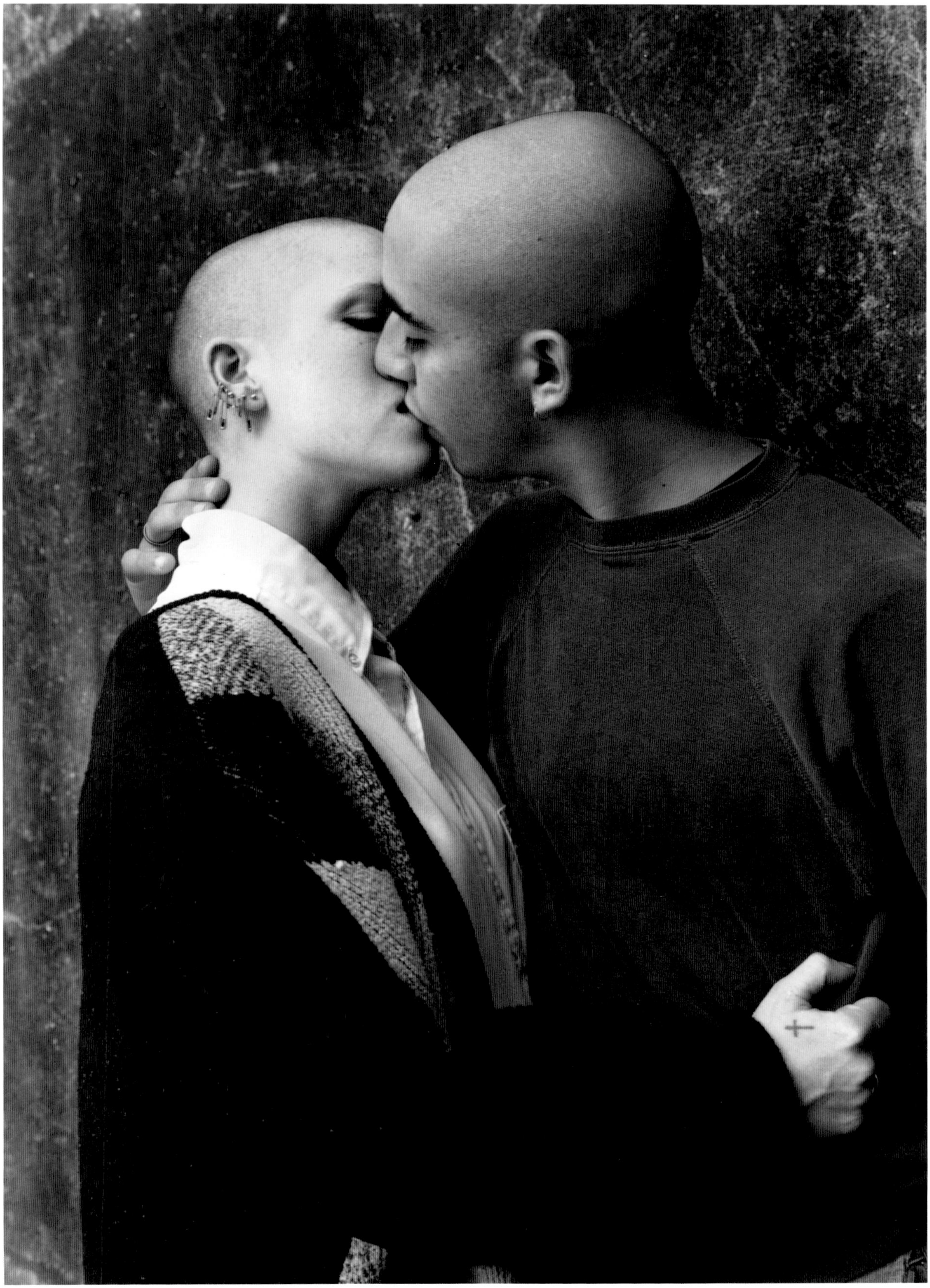

. . . If you ask me, said Marisa . . . it should be illegal for white people to have abortions, except in cases of incest or rape or birth defects, and it should be mandatory for all half-breeds and mixed breeds to have an abortion after one child and I said uh huh and she said are you still with that Asian girl?

"Flowers in Your Hair"
THIRTEEN STORIES AND THIRTEEN EPIGRAPHS

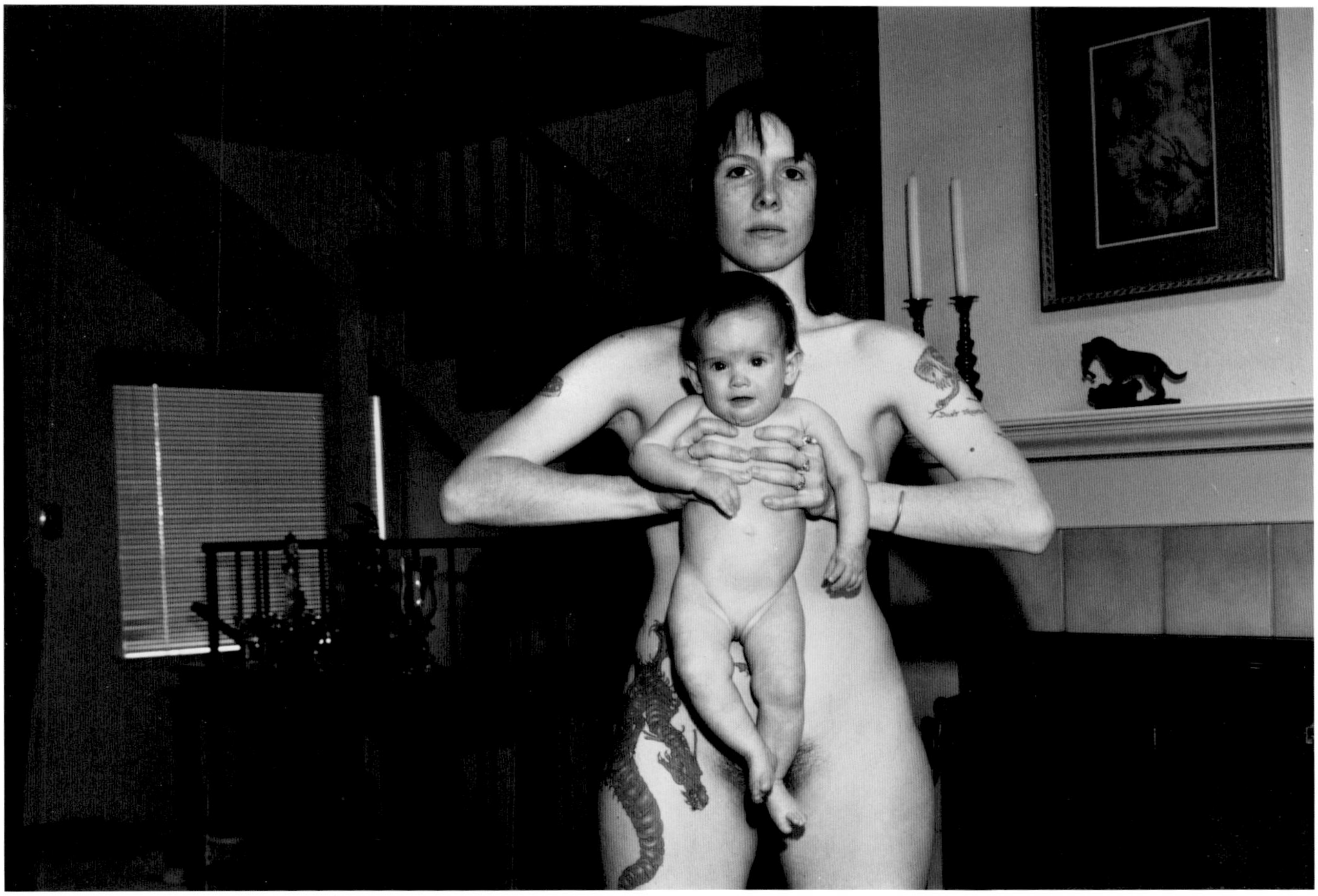

She had a very pretty oval head—I say head, not face, because hairlessness makes the boundary between head and face vanish so that there is only head, the cheeks and temples curving with inevitable naturalness around to the ears and back to the grey stubble (something other than hair) growing out from the bone. It was a finely colored head that Marisa had, clean and marbled like the freckled stone stairs fronting San Francisco houses.

"The White Knights"
THE RAINBOW STORIES

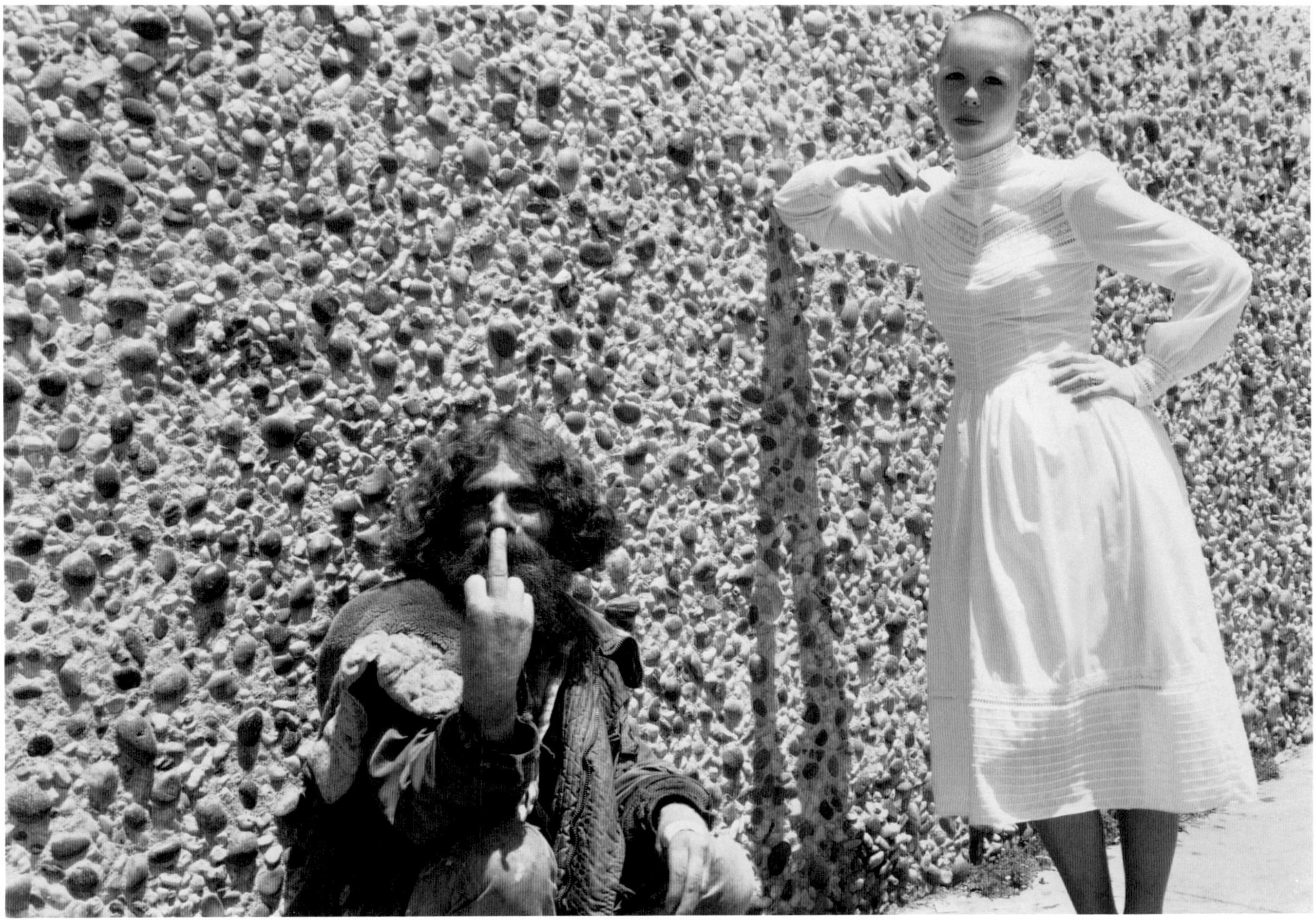

As to the future, either someone could arm and pay them (there are neo-Nazi camps in Germany and Austria, where boys practice being clean and orderly, with firearms training and mock executions to complete their education; there is a National Front in the U.K.; there is a Nazi printing company in Lincoln, Nebraska); or else they might get tired of being skinheads . . .

"The White Knights"
THE RAINBOW STORIES

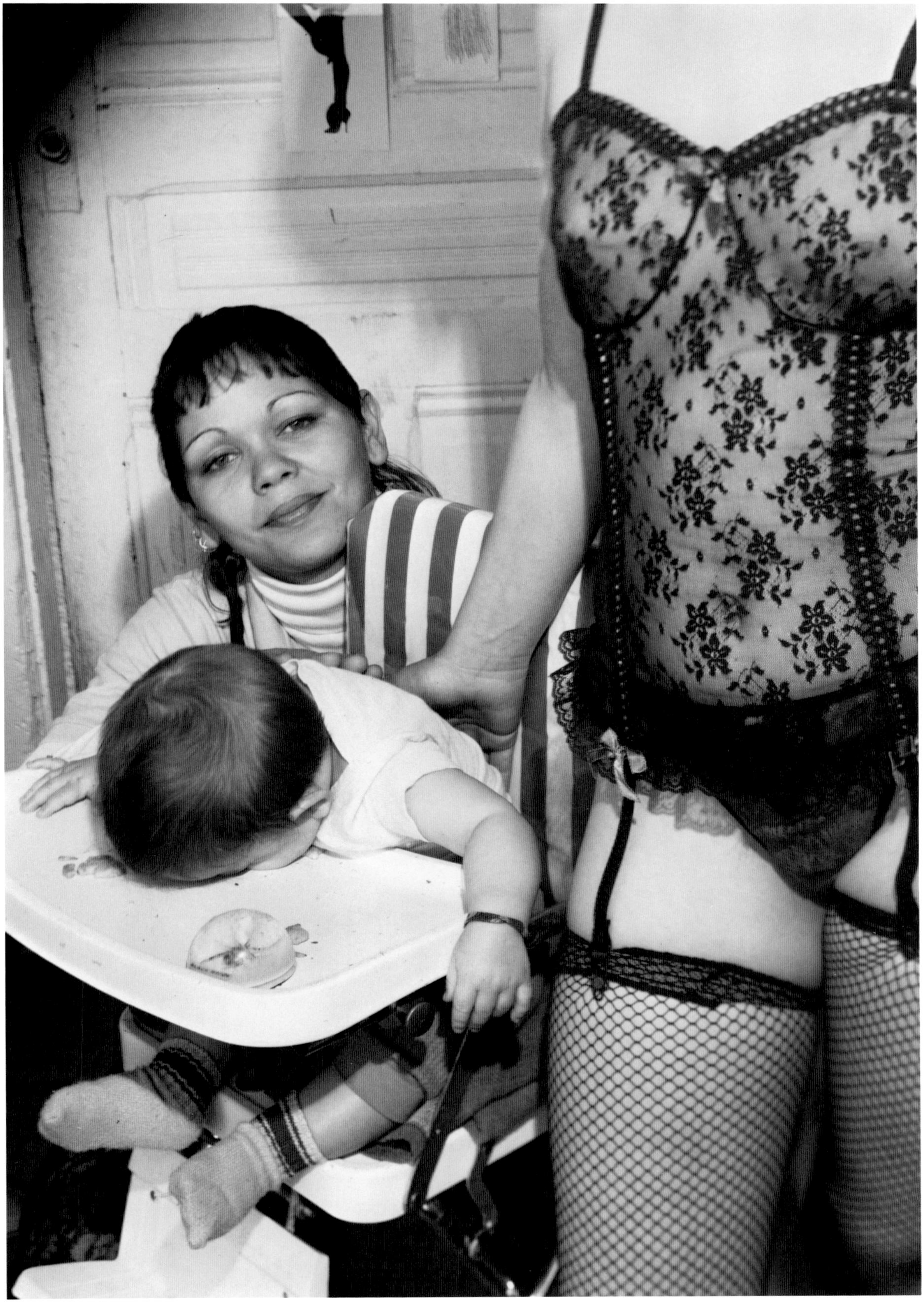

. . . but Korea really liked him as it seemed because she was strung out on speed and so she was sweet and serious with Jimmy (whores and undertakers are the only eternal optimists); and she said I *want* you I *need* you cause I'm a refugee from Korea so won't you come with me and Jimmy said baby maybe later and Korea said *no* we got to do it *now* cause at ten o'clock I got to be checked in at Saint Anthony's or else they'll be sending me back to Africa with all the other black, black people, but don't worry for yourself Jimmy babe cause you're so white that heaven's gonna come for you and if I'm good and get to know you and keep tricking for Christ I know you'll let me stay too and not be a refugee from Germany anymore cause my name is Berlin and Jimmy said I thought your name was Korea and Korea screamed now I can see you looking at me with those eyes of death.

WHORES FOR GLORIA

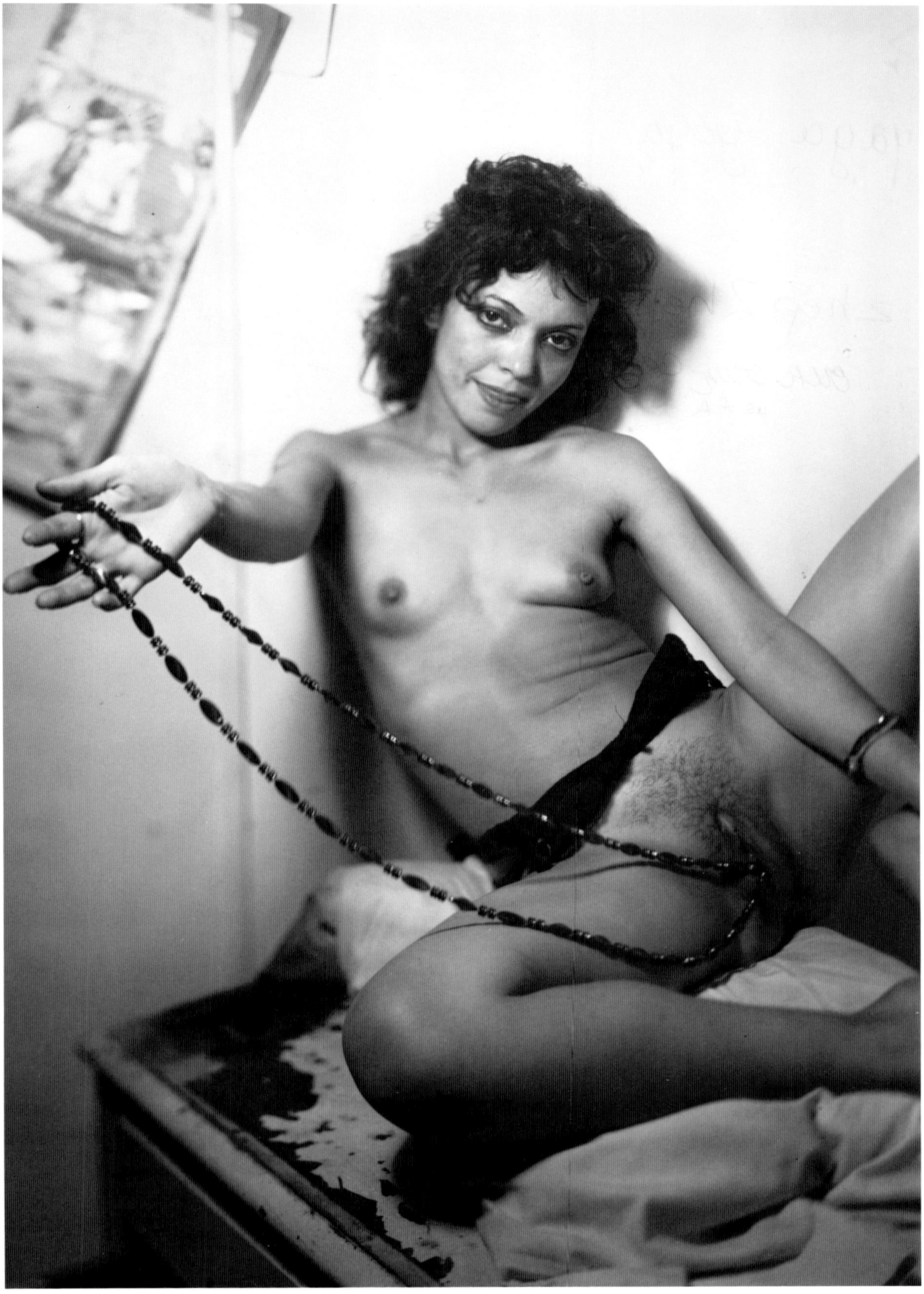

"It get boring," Tina sighed, "jumping into bed with every Tom, Dick and Harry."

"Have you ever had anyone you were in love with?"

"Once, but I had a lot of men in love with me." She chuckled. "And I taken *advantage* of it."

"Ladies and Red Lights"
THE RAINBOW STORIES

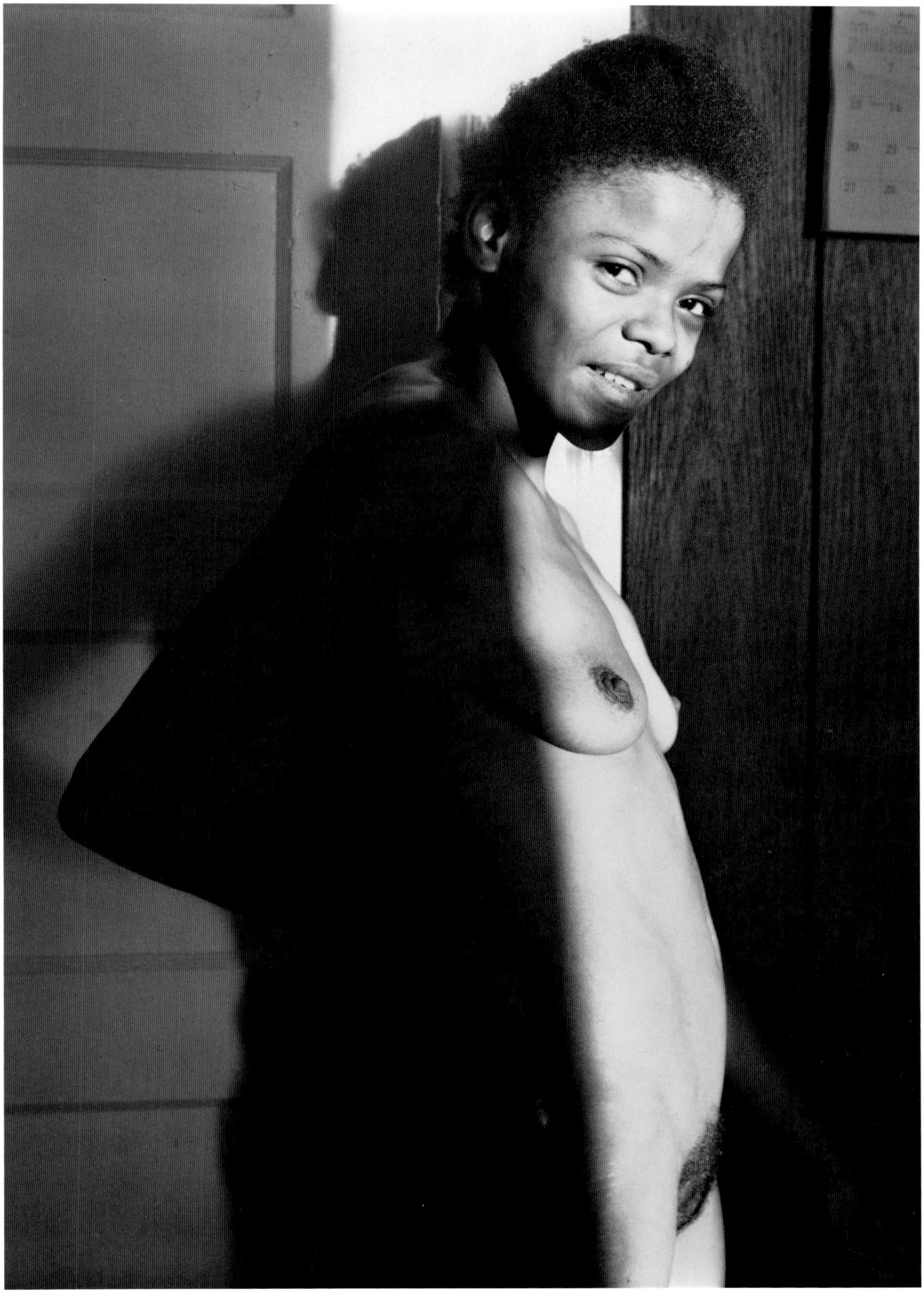

So I says look I can give you your money back there's no problem here. I can walk home or something. I really don't need this date to the point where I'm gonna get hurt if that's what it's gonna take to satisfy you. He says you know I just want some head and if you're good enough you're not gonna get hurt. Well luckily I'm real good at that. But all the time I was servicing him I was in fear. So when I finished servicing him yeah I could tell that he was checking out where his diamond rings and things were, so I didn't get nowhere *near* 'em, so I says are you done with me now he says *yes* I'm *done* here's a dollar for bus fare. Well I'm not gonna argue with him I'm not gonna say *oh,* you're not gonna bring me back? I didn't do that. I was pretty shook to where I just walked. You know I'm a pretty good judge of character and you really have to watch out the look they have and the way they drool.

WHORES FOR GLORIA

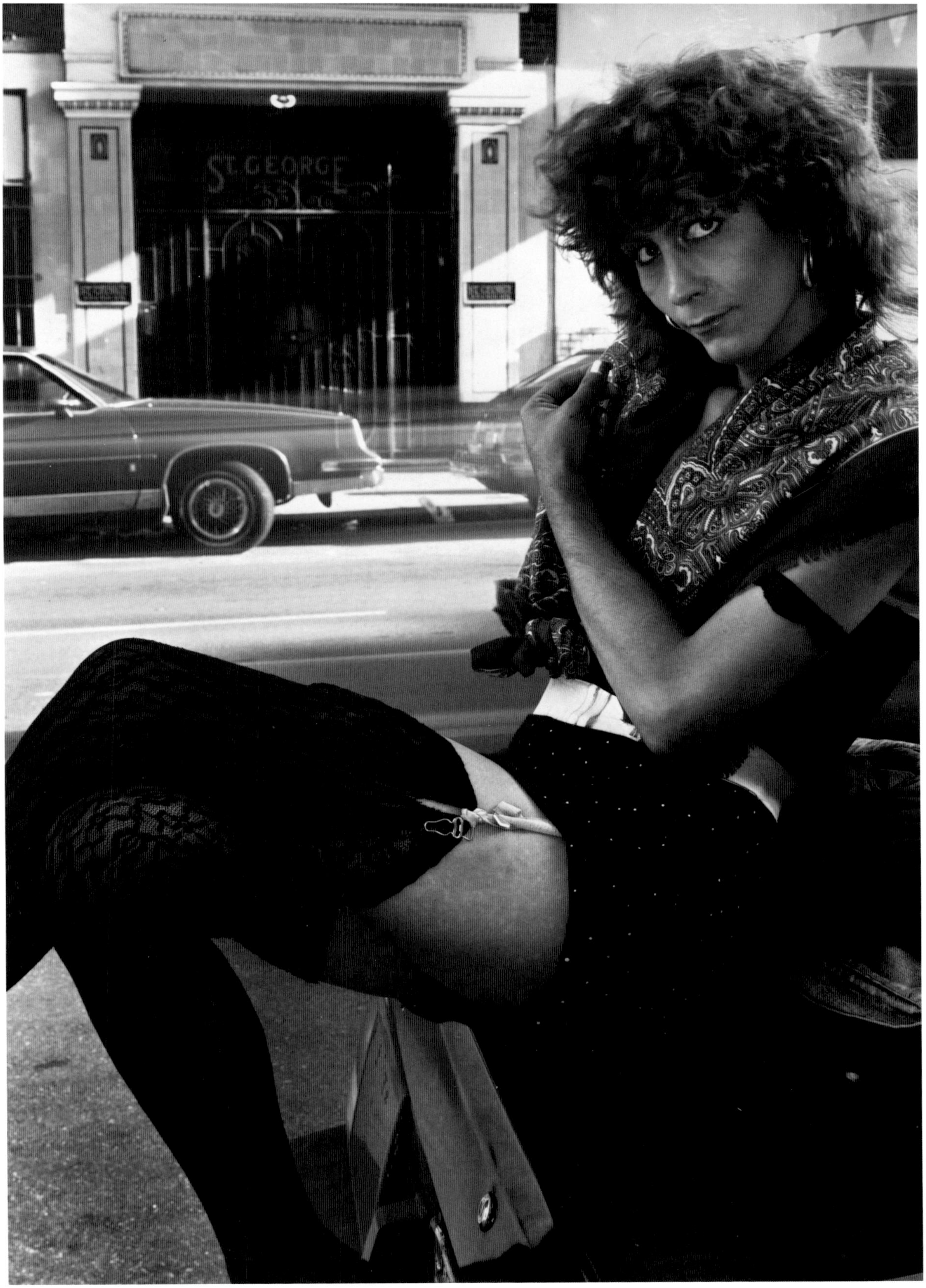
St. GEORGE

Oy sat by the water jug and waggled her tongue at imaginary customers again . . . It was Thanksgiving behind the mirror.

"The Happy Girls"
Thirteen Stories and Thirteen Epigraphs

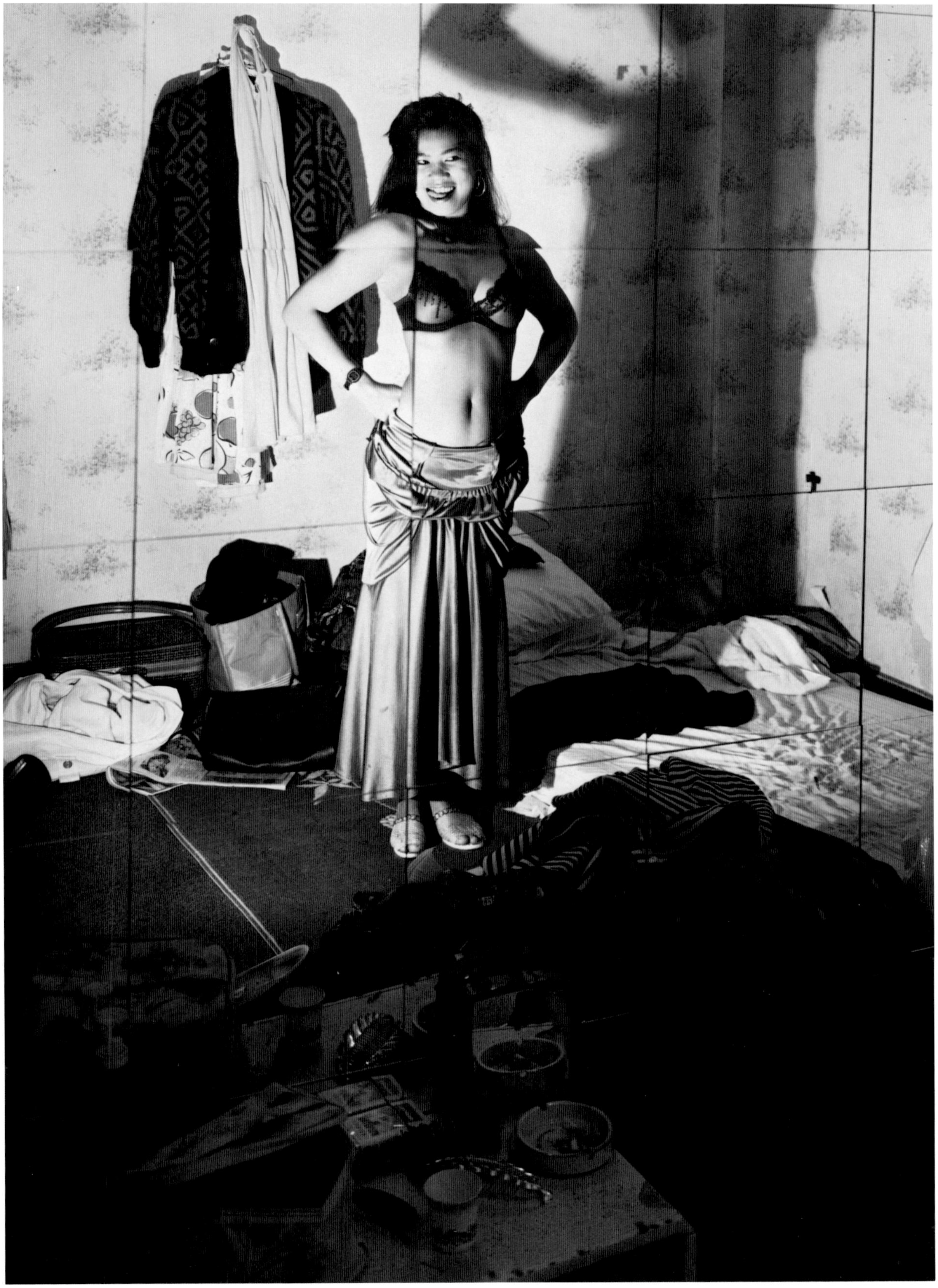

On one of those days when at two in the afternoon it was still morning because Jimmy had woken up with the dry heaves and the thought of a beer almost gave him the wet heaves, so he was sitting in the Black Rose drinking watery orange juice and nasty tomato juice and a whore came up to ask him for a quarter to do her laundry and it was more of an effort to get rid of her than to give her the quarter and the electronic sign-strip over the video screen said CECILY – CECILY – CECILY and Cecily stood behind the bar and said Hey, baby to Jimmy softly when he came in and he was not sure whether he had been there a long time or whether he had just gotten there.

WHORES FOR GLORIA

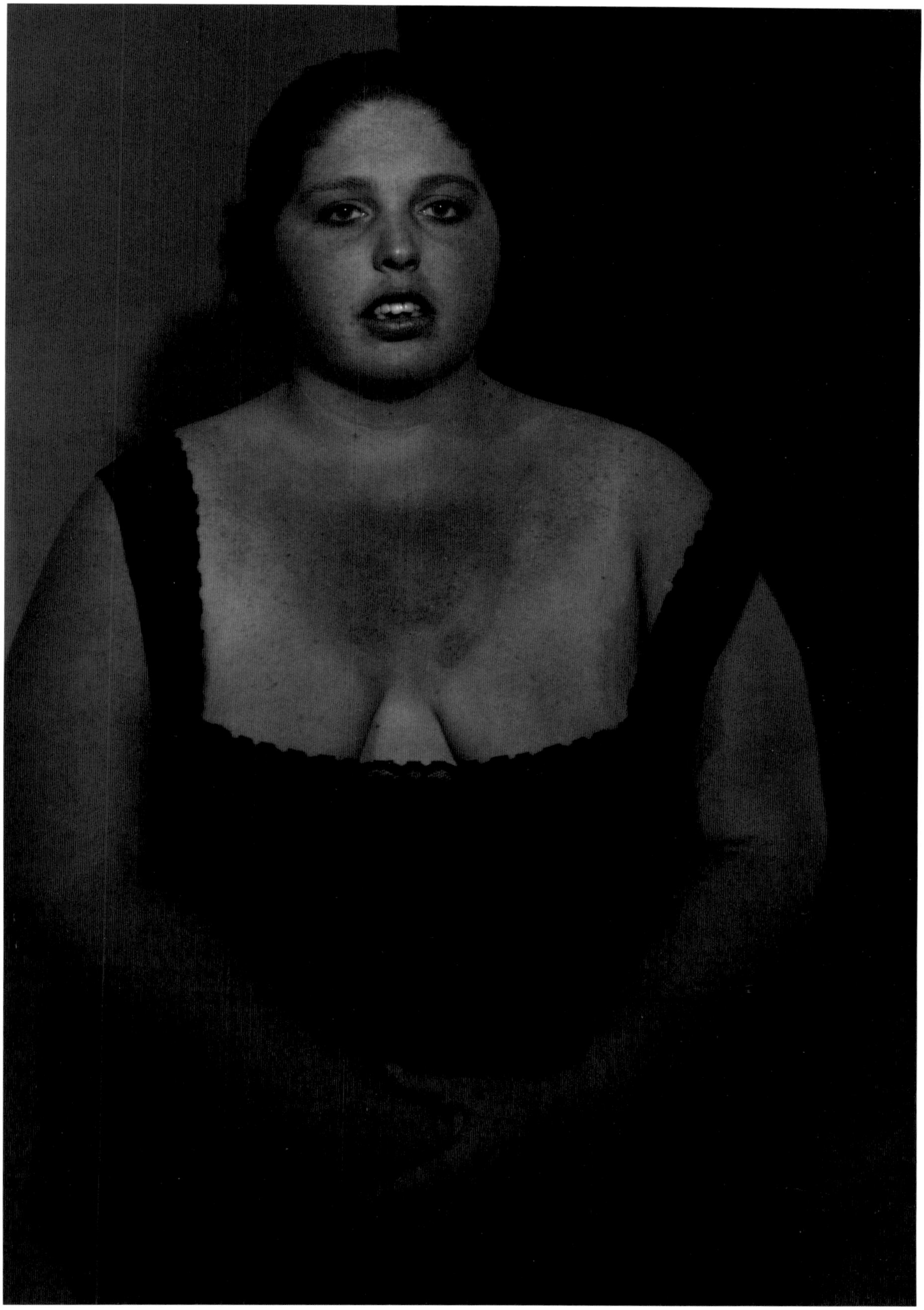

Yes, it was a sunny happy day, happy as a whore down on hands and knees to make you laugh in the doorway of a hotel, wiggling her shiny satin ass, and the laces of the whateveritwas dug into her flanks going back and forth like bootstrings, funny as the doggishly ugly faces of fortyish transvestite whores pursing their cheeks and loudly wolf-whistling at men whom they thought might just might want to have their dicks sucked, transvestite whores alone or in pairs or even in threes playfully slapping each other's paunches with fat arms, showing off their hormone tits with winks and calls and looks from side to side to make sure that Laredo and the other undercover bitches weren't rolling down the street in a van or an old junker that tried so hard not to look anything like the standard black-and-white that had busted and would bust every last one of them, over and over, confiscating their money when they caught them in the act.

WHORES FOR GLORIA

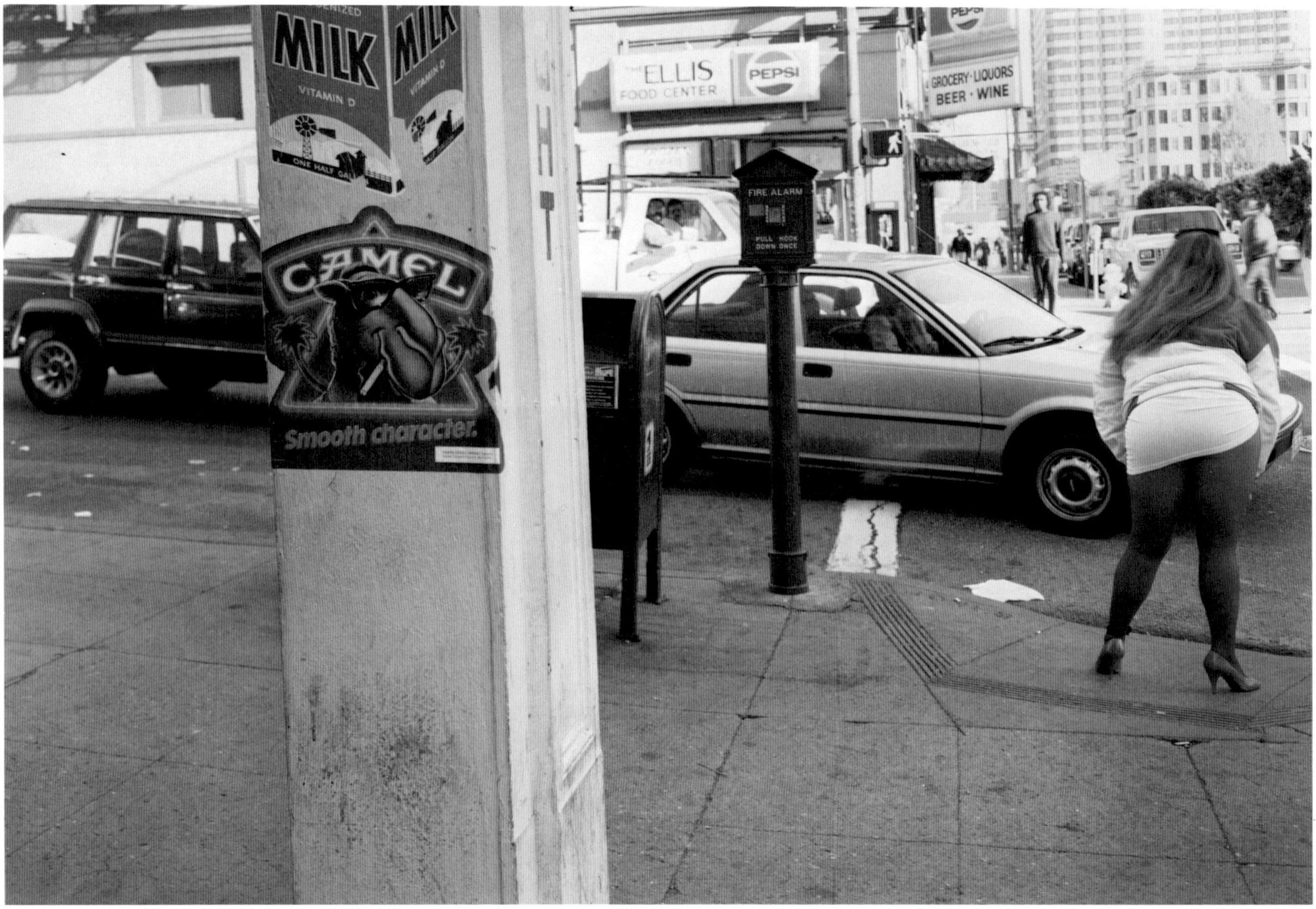
MILK
VITAMIN D
ELLIS
FOOD CENTER
PEPSI
GROCERY · LIQUORS
BEER · WINE
FIRE ALARM
PULL HOOK
DOWN ONCE
CAMEL
Smooth character.

"I like comfort," he explained. "I'm not that concerned with looking like a woman.—Oh, *where's* my black bra?"

THE ICE-SHIRT

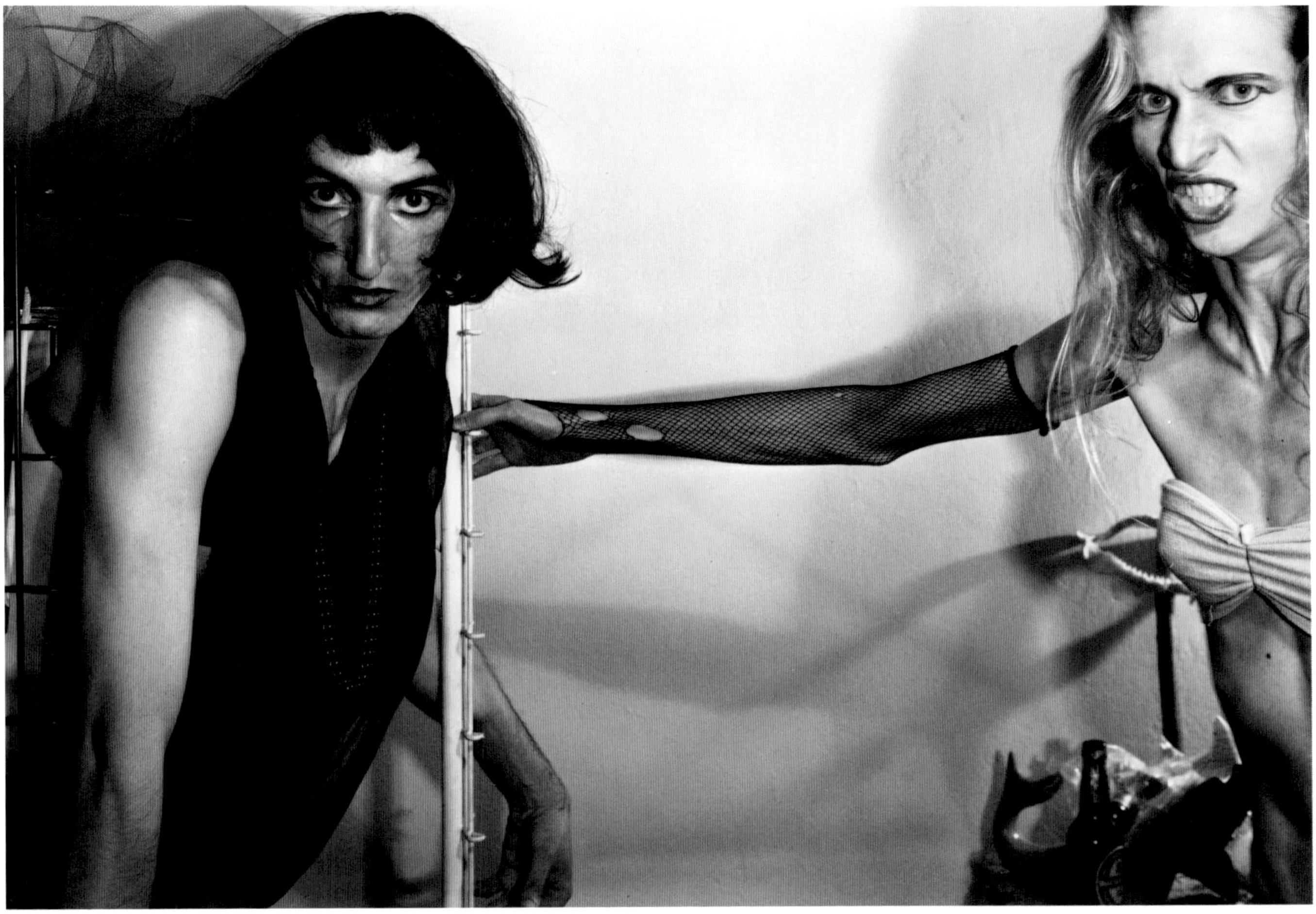

Jack looked great, although he had scars. He didn't have junky ways. He just had a 3-c.c. syringe. Every morning he woke up to something like morning sickness and had to get his speedball right away, but *he* wasn't addicted. If he didn't shoot up, on the first day his body would say all *right* you motherfucker I'm gonna GET you, but on the second day he would be OVER it, man; he would be healthy as pie.

WHORES FOR GLORIA

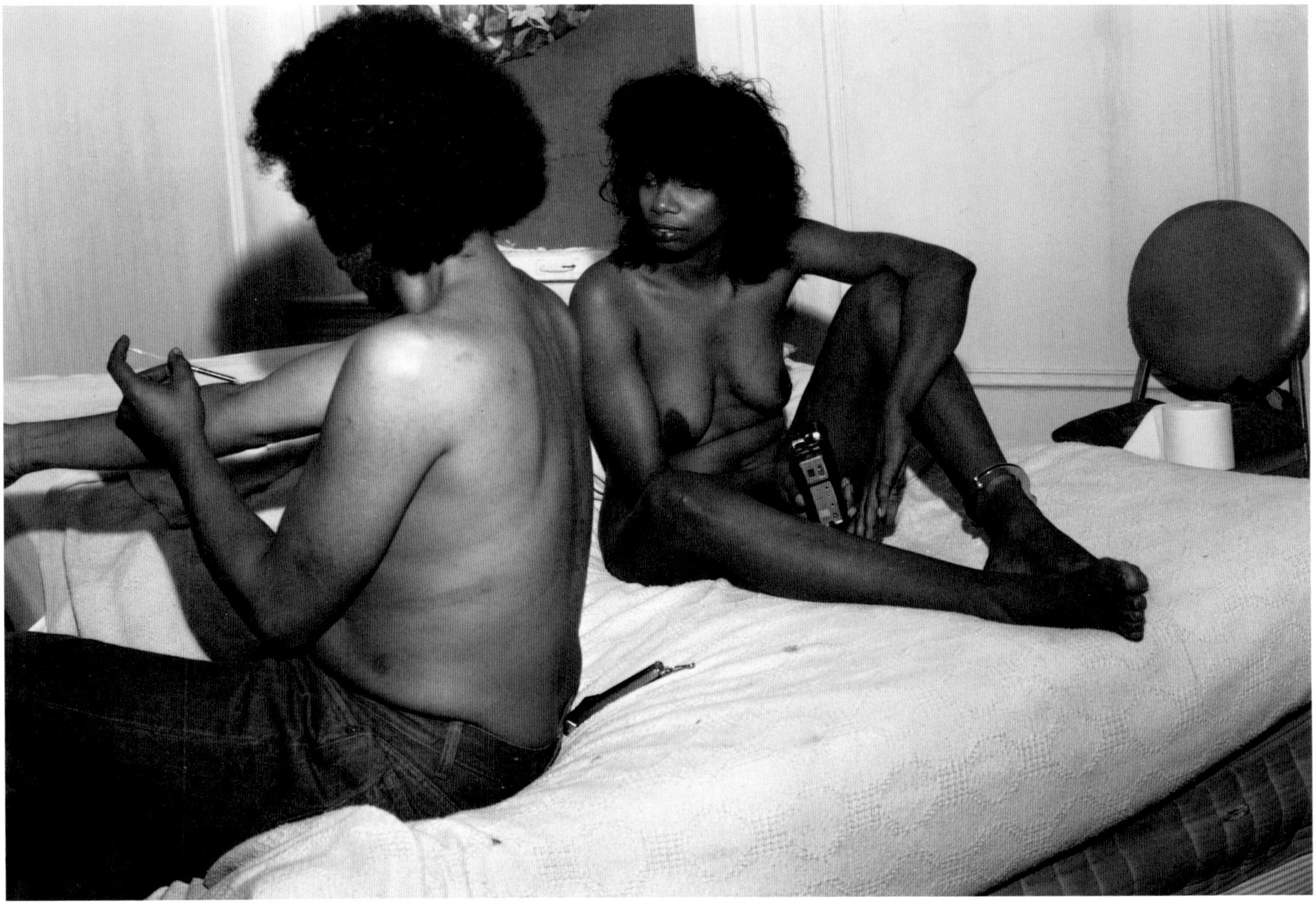

Keiko's arms were not just scarred but lined, patched, painted and folded with purple scars. Her face was serene. I remembered her glistening eyes; her hair, originally cold Asian black, dyed brown, but greying at the roots, her buttocks flabby and scarred in ovals like bruises, her face suddenly stiff and weary, her breasts hanging down so wearily when she lay on her side to be sexy with what she called her "sleepy look."

"Flowers in Your Hair"
THIRTEEN STORIES AND THIRTEEN EPIGRAPHS

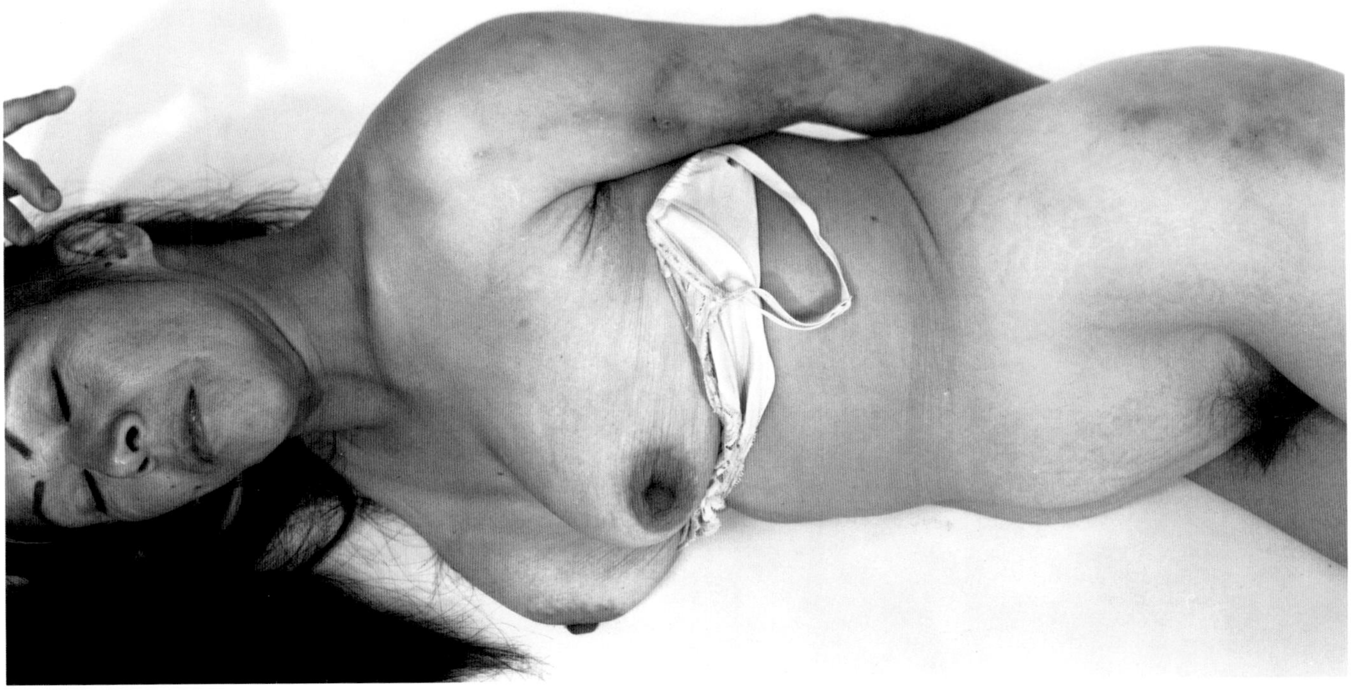

. . . and old people hobbled home to their hotels to double-lock their half-rotten doors for the night and it got darker and the whores came out and sat on the hoods of old station wagons and Laredo spied on them with all-seeing eyes of a snorkeler . . .

Whores for Gloria

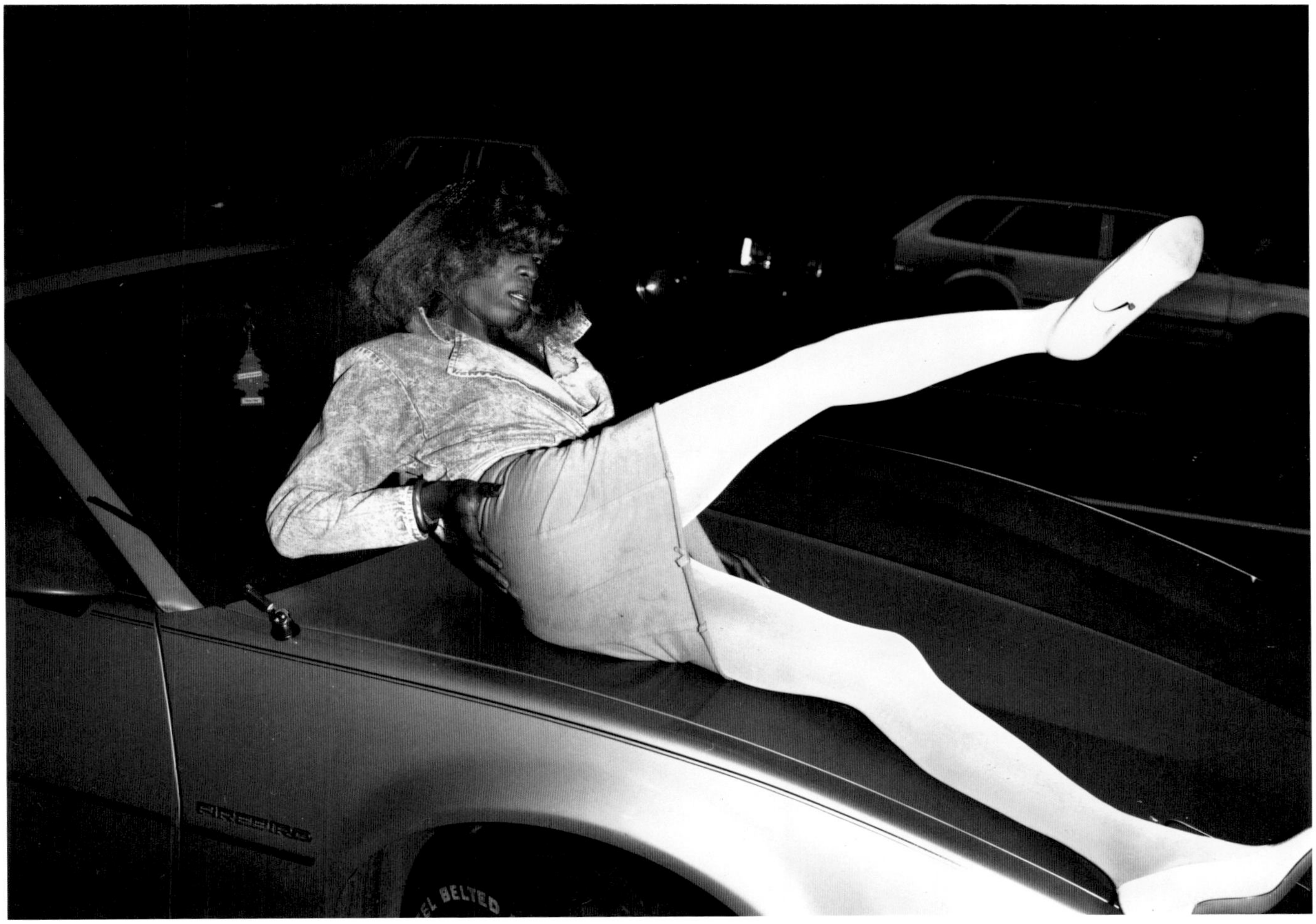
FIREBIRD
BELTED

—How divinely diminutive my dress would be if there were no flesh and stubborn bone to keep her from maximizing her minimalization.—

THE RAINBOW STORIES

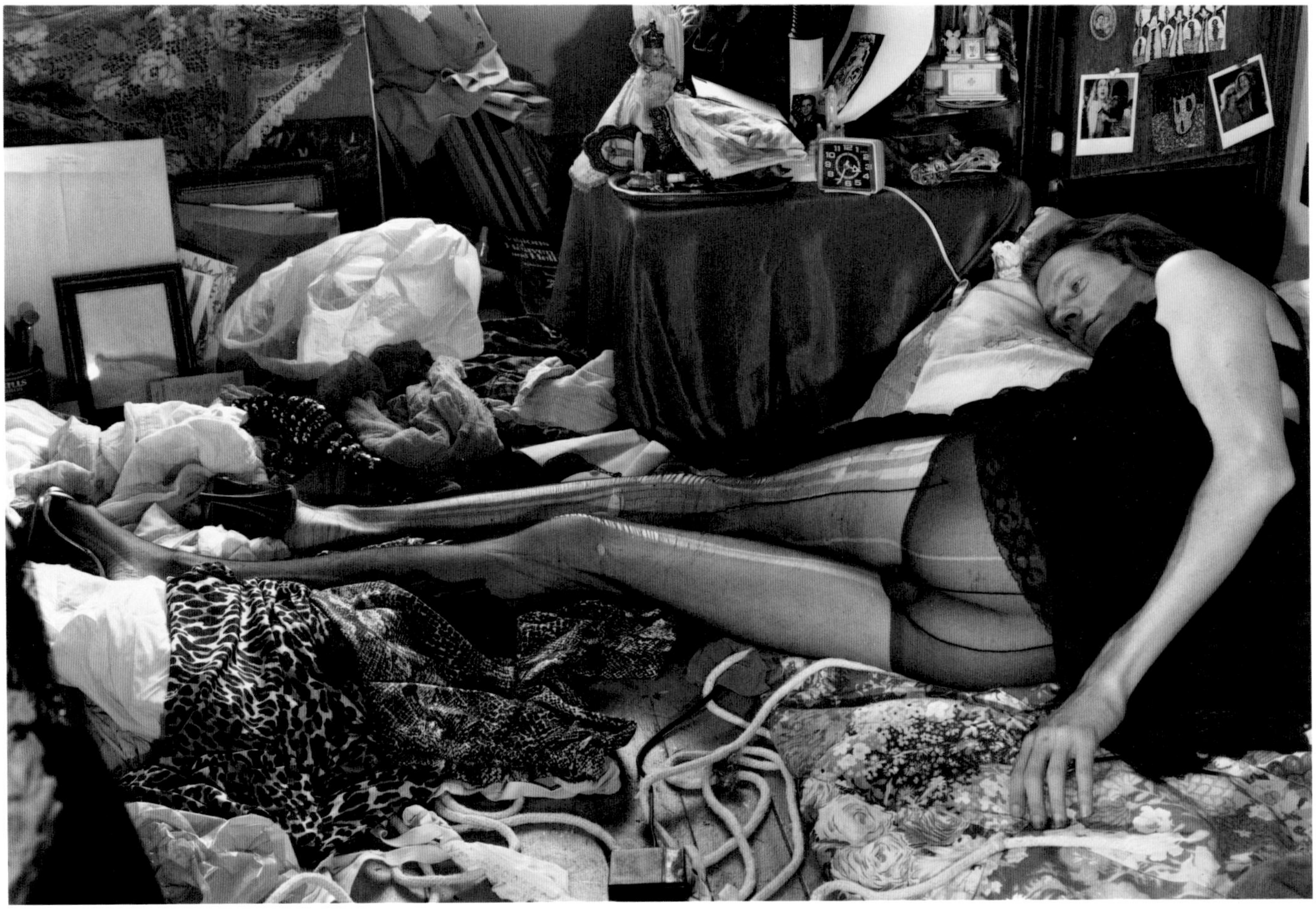

I had this one Kung Fu master that loved to be my slave, laughed Dinah, yawning and stretching her body like a snake, scratching herself, lying naked on the bed with Jimmy's stiletto between her legs. —And he liked for me to tie him up and choke him around the neck, then make him suck my *toes* and things. And he wrote me out a contract for his life. —Dinah giggled. —And he said I could do whatever I wanted to do to him. I could rent 'im out to my friends an' I could beat 'im, and if he happened to die—*huh!*—he had my permission. I mean, I had his permission. I had this other date; he looked just like Kenny Rogers. And he would like for me to give 'im golden showers. He liked for me to drink like a sixpack of beer and then after about a good hour then he'd want me to piss all in his mouth and he'd gobble it down just as fast as I could piss it out.

WHORES FOR GLORIA

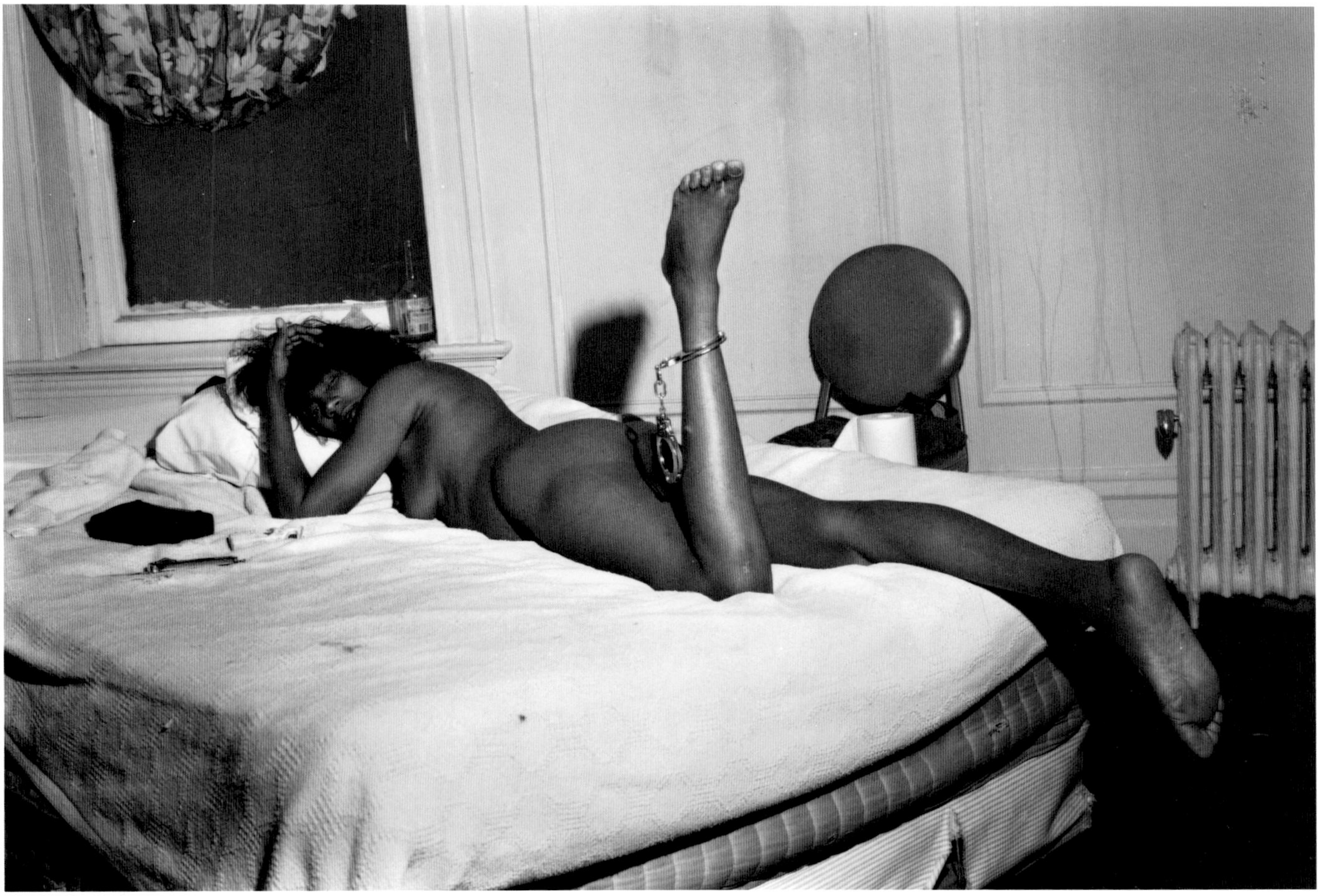

The Wrecking Crew hid from the wind, wrapped in dirty blankets and dirty coats and dirty foam pads. They had hoarse voices. — "Evangeline, gimme a cigarette!" said He-Wolf. — Ease up on that," goes old Evangeline, with her round red face and grey hair bobbing angrily like a fishing-float in a stream.

"The Blue Yonder"
THE RAINBOW STORIES

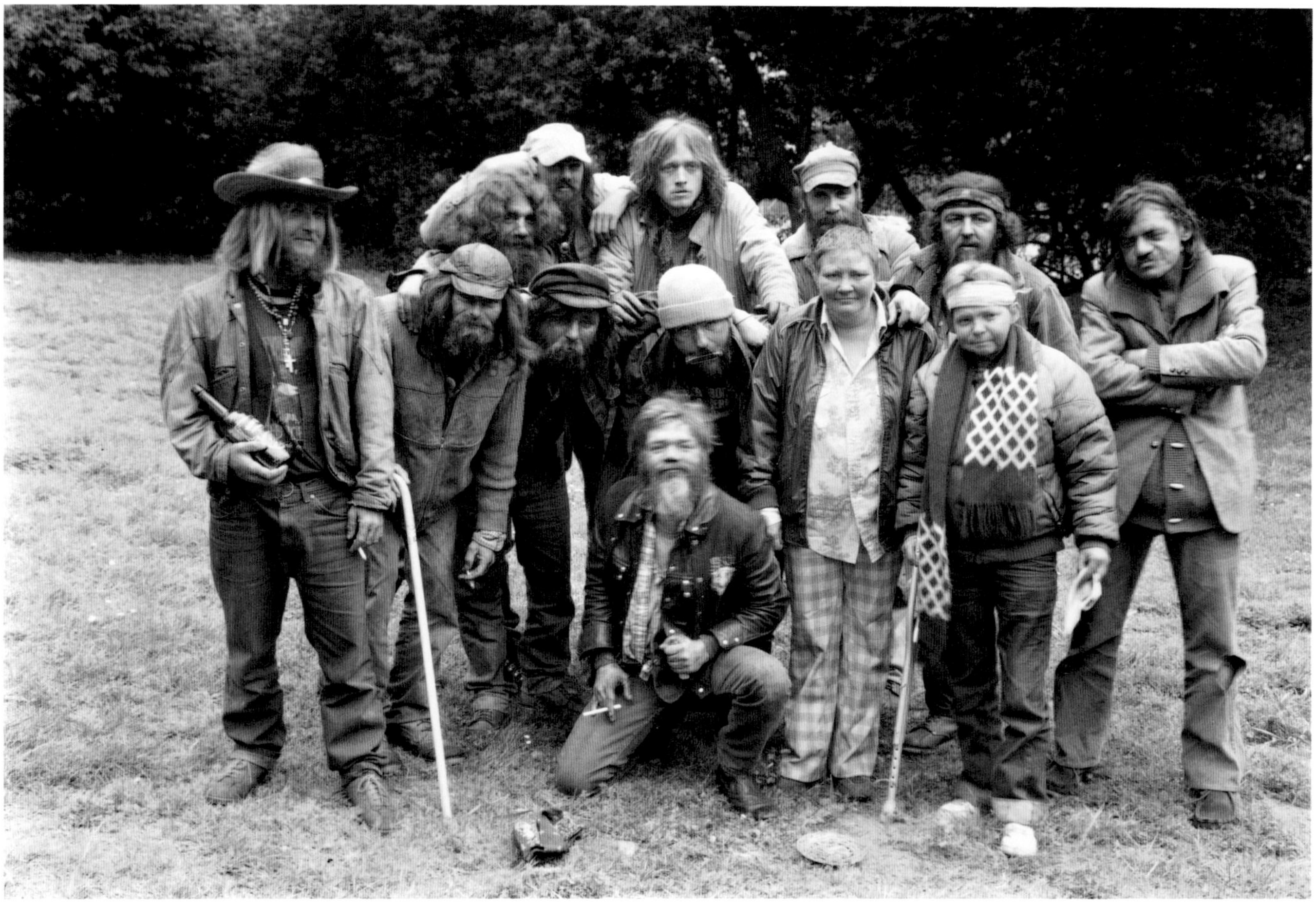

For five minutes he groaned and fumbled slowly with his boots. Suddenly the darkness was permeated by a stench compounded of sweat, toenails and turning vinegar.

"The Blue Yonder"
THE RAINBOW STORIES

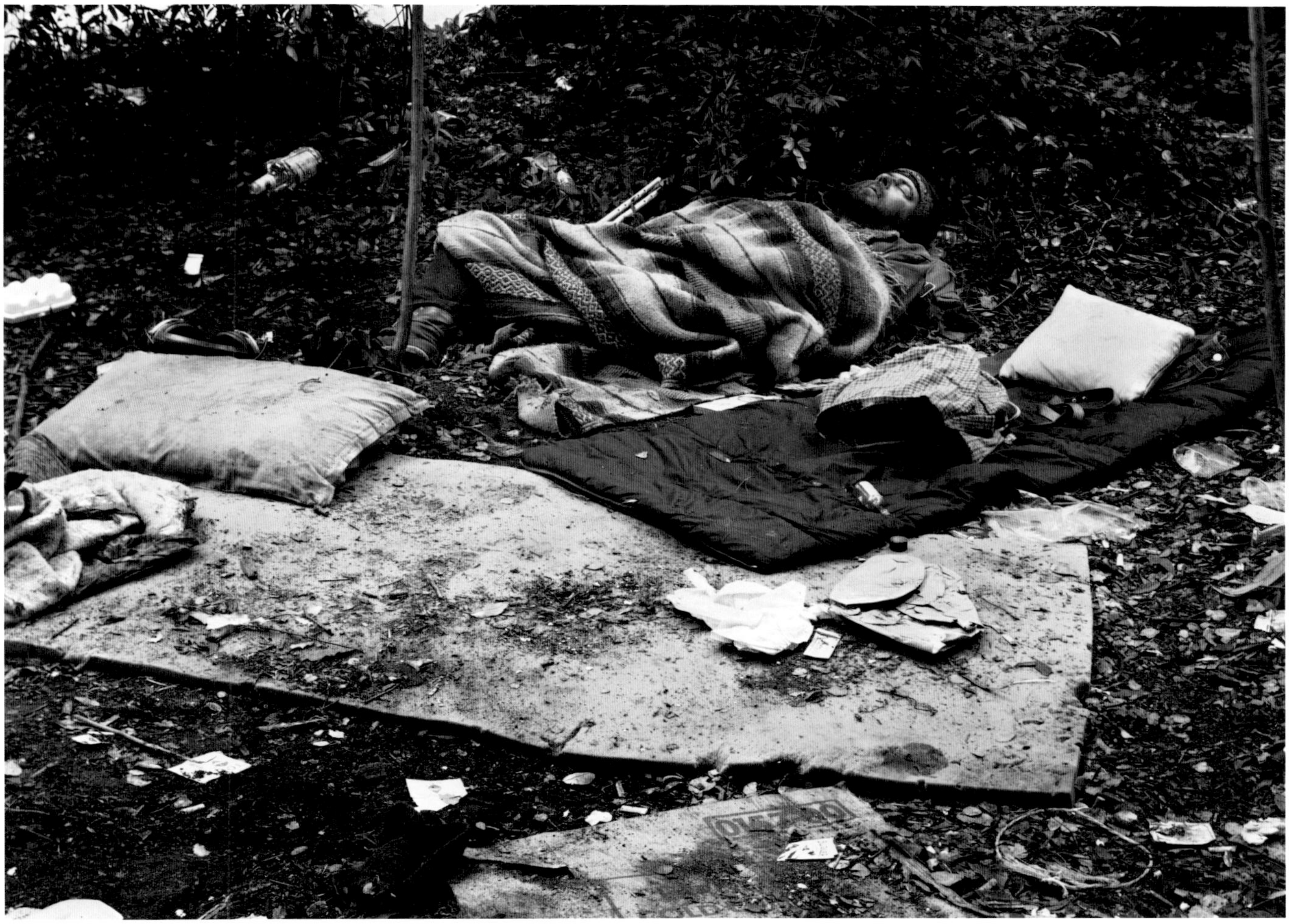

Awright, Now, the first thing is ya see, I useta wanna be something, only here I am, just a lousy drunk. You don't haveta tell me I'm a drunk. I know I'm a drunk. Are you tryin to tell me I'm a drunk?

"Flowers in your Hair"
THIRTEEN STORIES AND THIRTEEN EPITAPHS

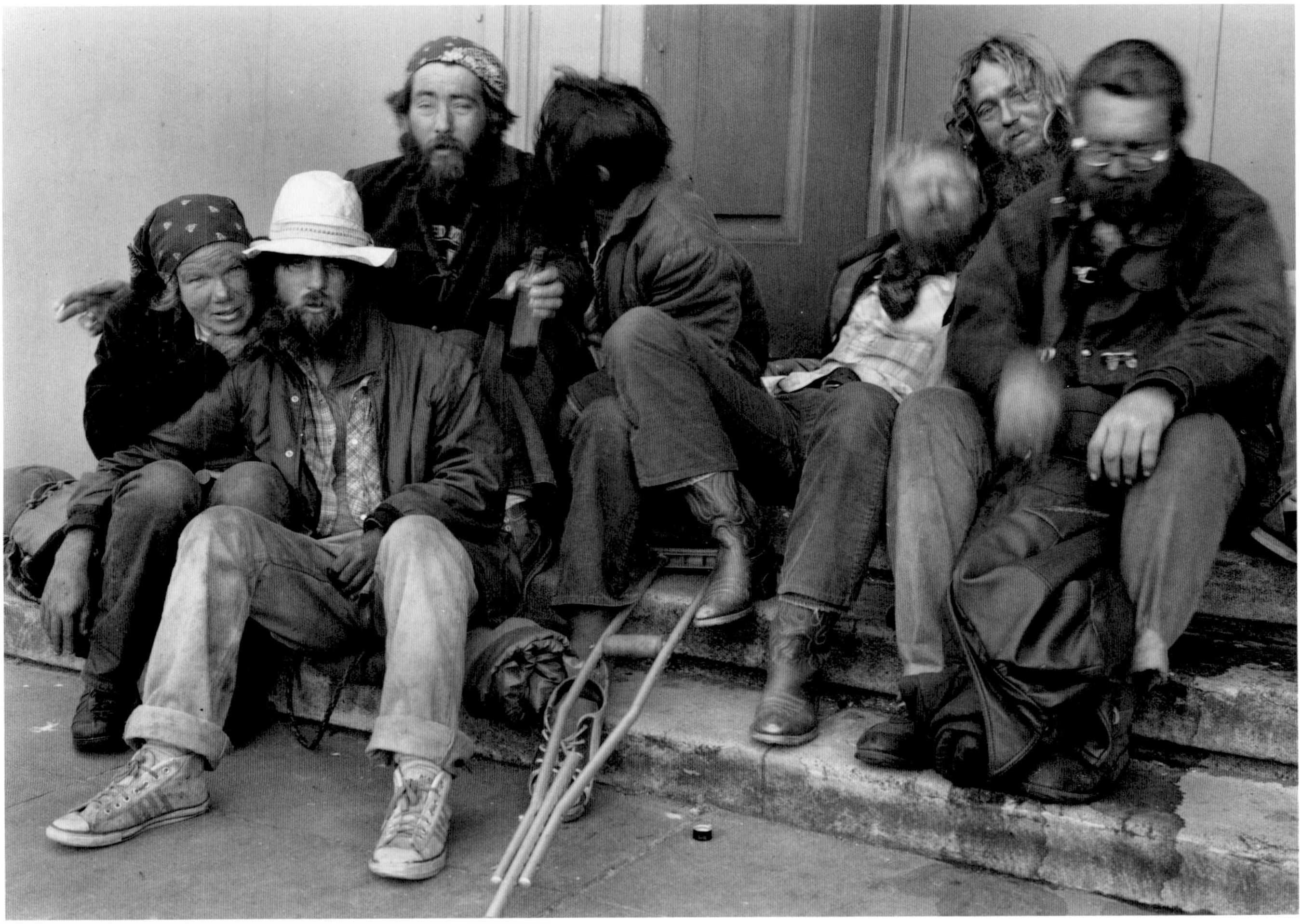

"I think He-Wolf's gone to Seattle," said Rich, and that may have been true. "He said he had an itch to get out of here." That was why nobody ever saw him again.

"The Blue Yonder"
THE RAINBOW STORIES

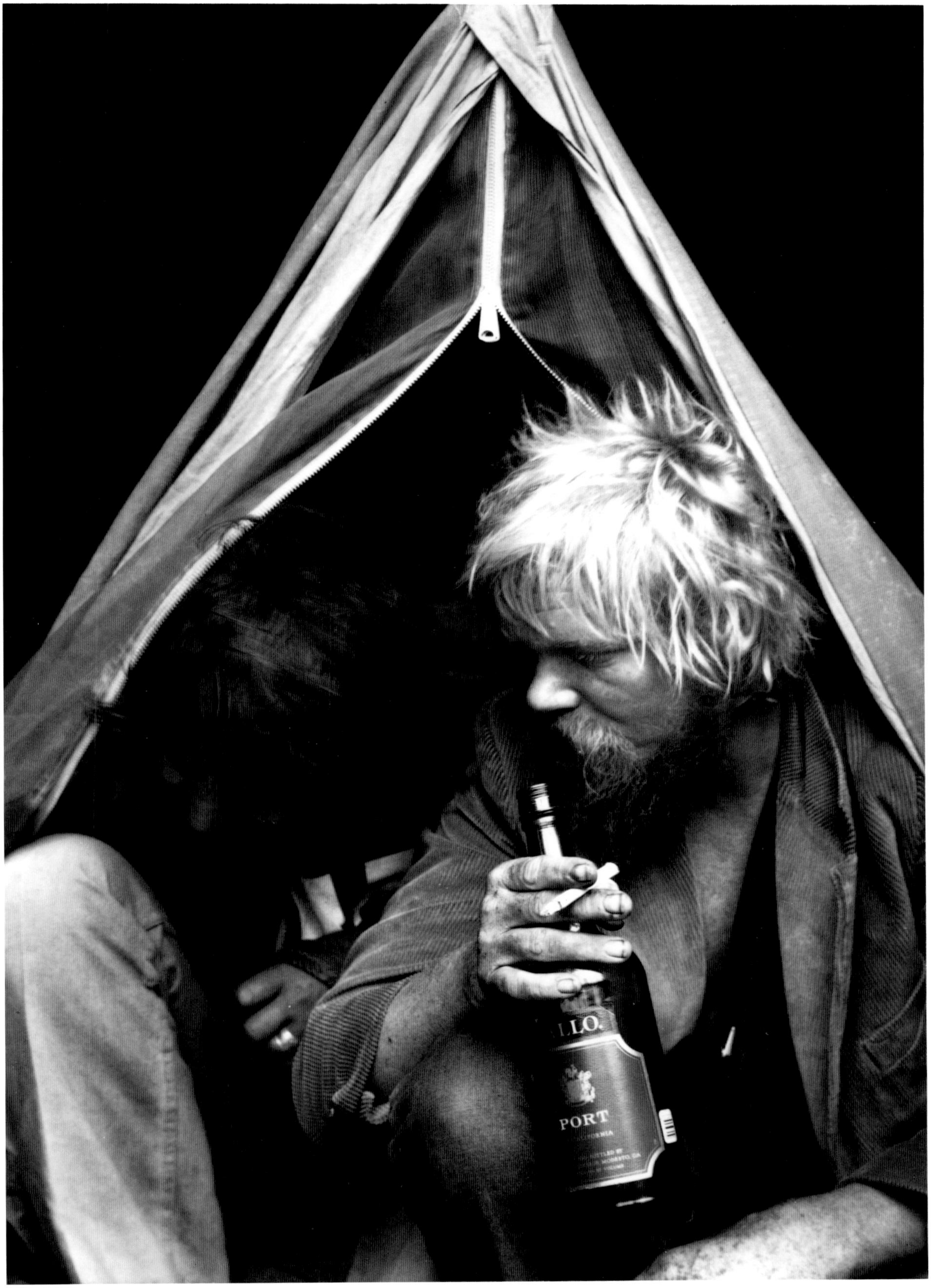
PORT

. . . Laddie sat thinking so that his head rose like a cloud of white beard and white locks above his cowboy hands that rolled joints without him: and his irises seemed to spiral inward in continuation of the trios of wrinkles at eye-corners that hooked out like rays . . .

"Kindness"
THIRTEEN STORIES AND THIRTEEN EPIGRAPHS

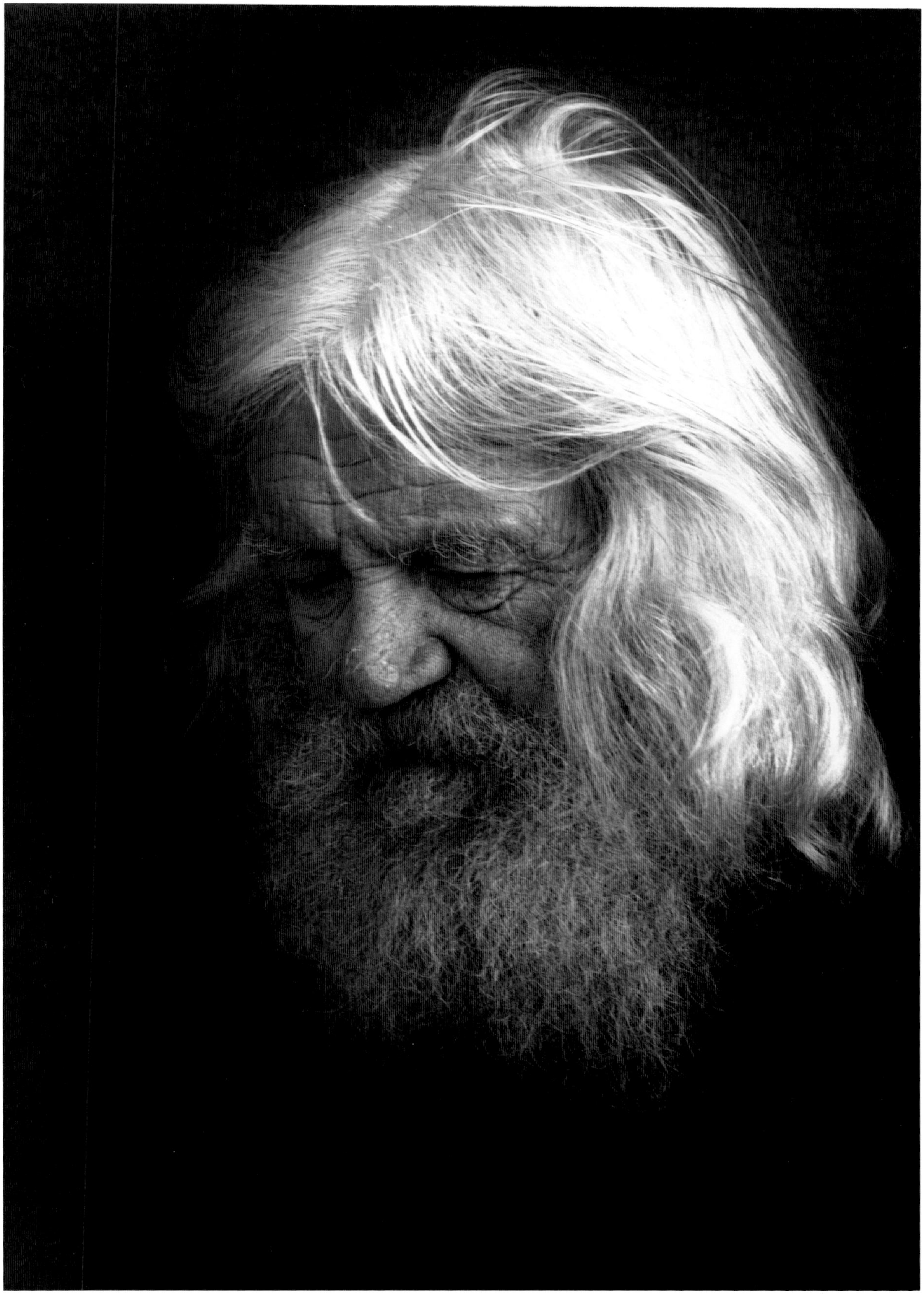

"I read the newspapers this morning," confessed Cory Smith. "You know, I always like to look at the obituary page, just like Mr. Baumeister. You see, Mr. Baumeister knows everybody that *ever* died!"

"The Blue Yonder"
THE RAINBOW STORIES

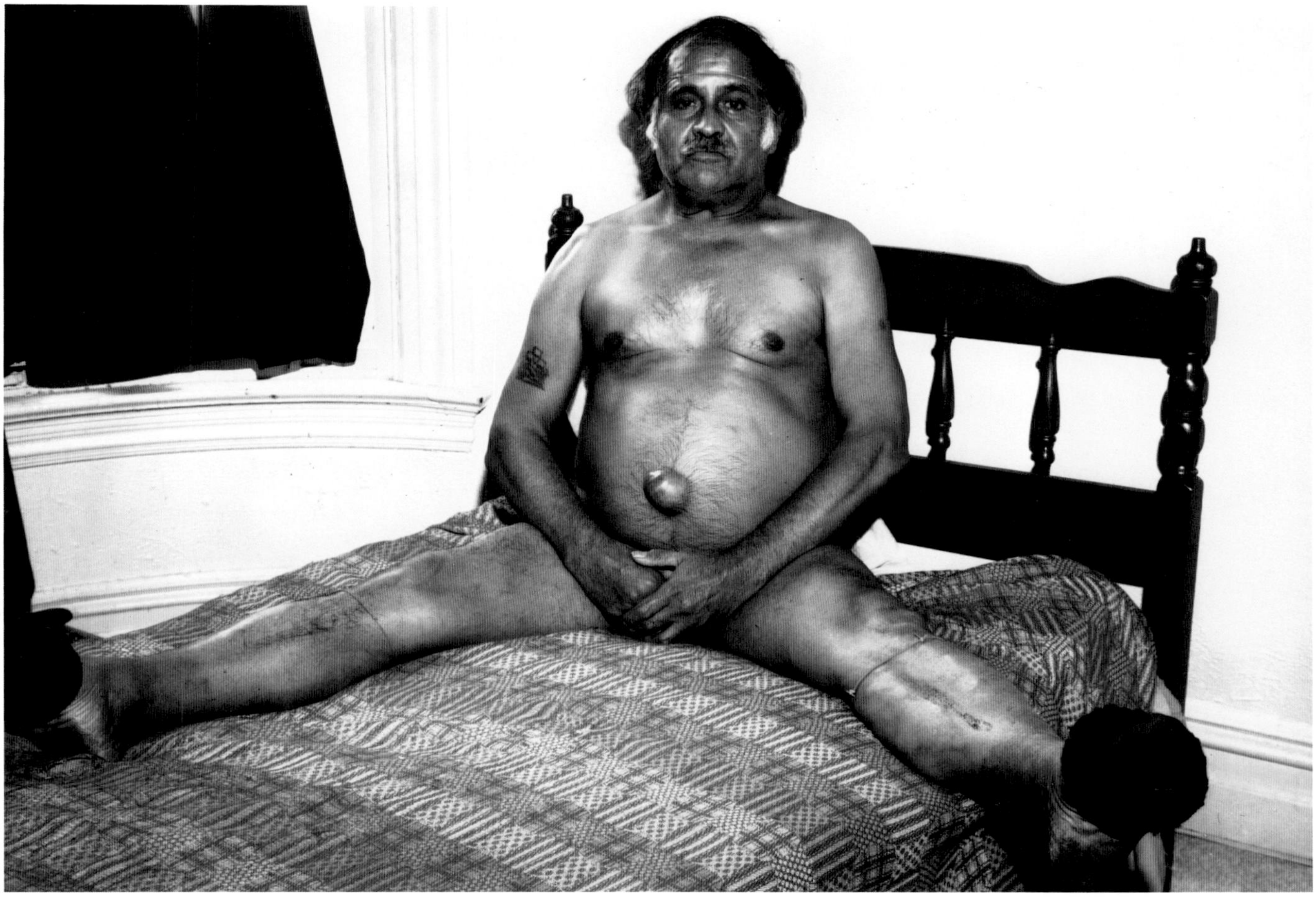

She lived uneasily among the Boarding Care Men, who leaned in their TV chairs and glared at the blue screen with eyes as brightly sullen as stars about to shoot down, down into the blue atmosphere . . .

"The Blue Yonder"
THE RAINBOW STORIES

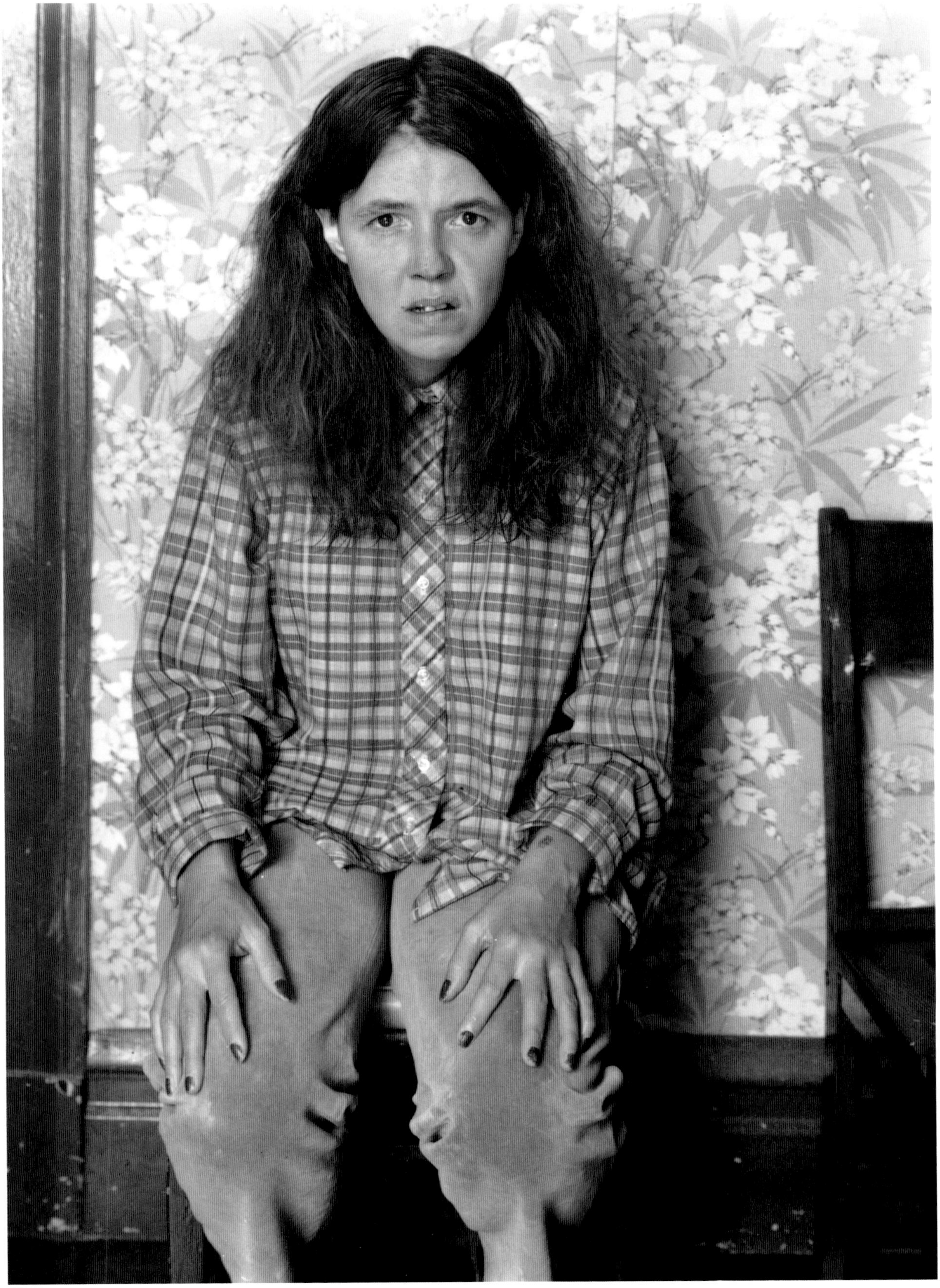

When you get drunken crushes on women whose drunken mothers used to try to stab them: when the names of streets are like Nabokov's wearisome cleverness; when only the pretty shapes of women have integrity and when you close your eyes still see them leaning and crossing their legs and milking their tits at you, THEN you may on occasion like Jimmy find yourself looking down a long black block, down the tunnels of infinity to a streetlamp, a corner and a woman's waiting silhouette. – Or else like Jimmy you may have another drink.

WHORES FOR GLORIA

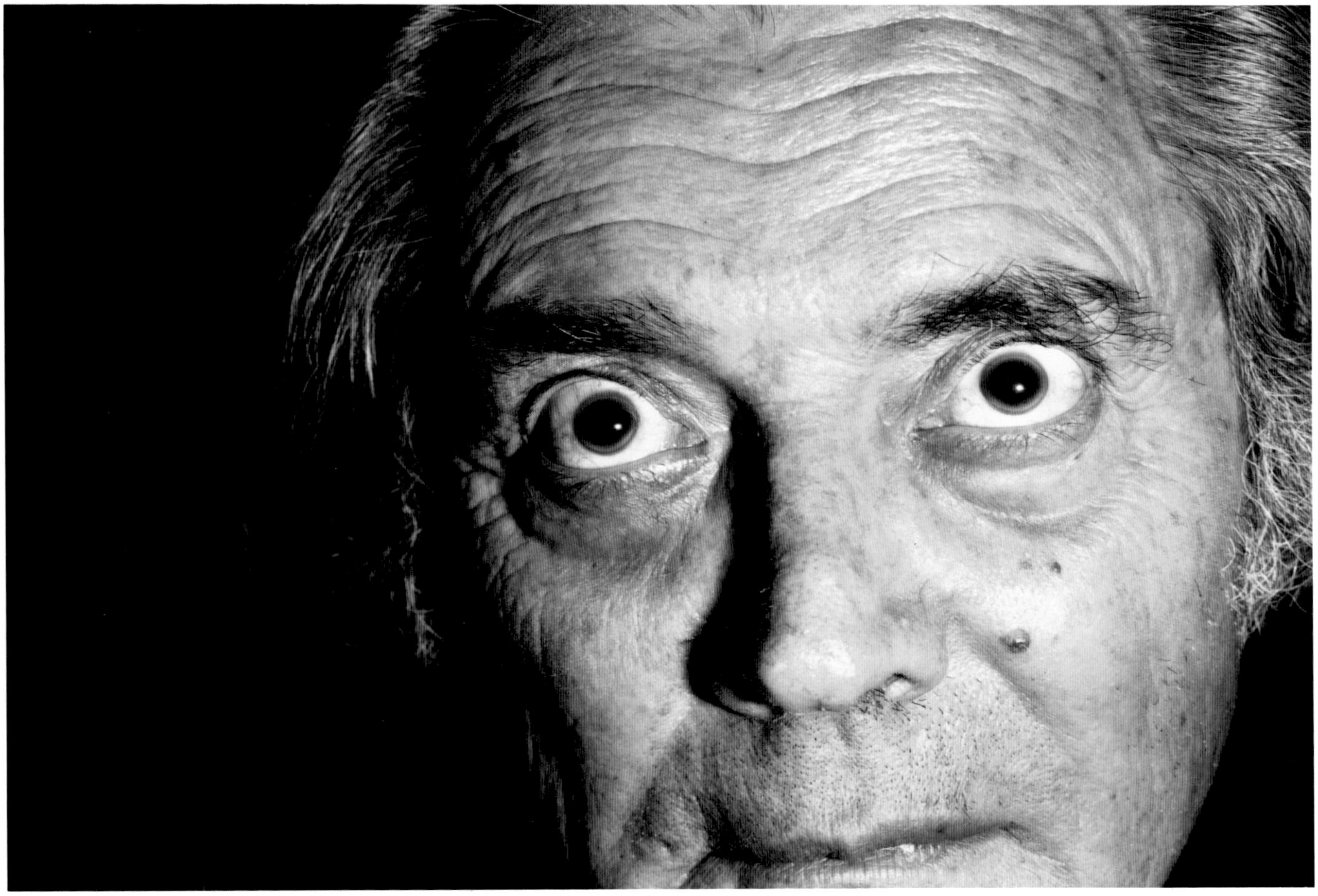

Phyllis got busted, too—for smack. No one knew who'd snitched on her. Linda, Luna and Fawn moved out of the Hotel Canada. Linda & Fawn got busted or left town; no one saw them anymore. Luna moved to the Paradise Hotel.

Phyllis and her Friend
WHORES FOR GLORIA

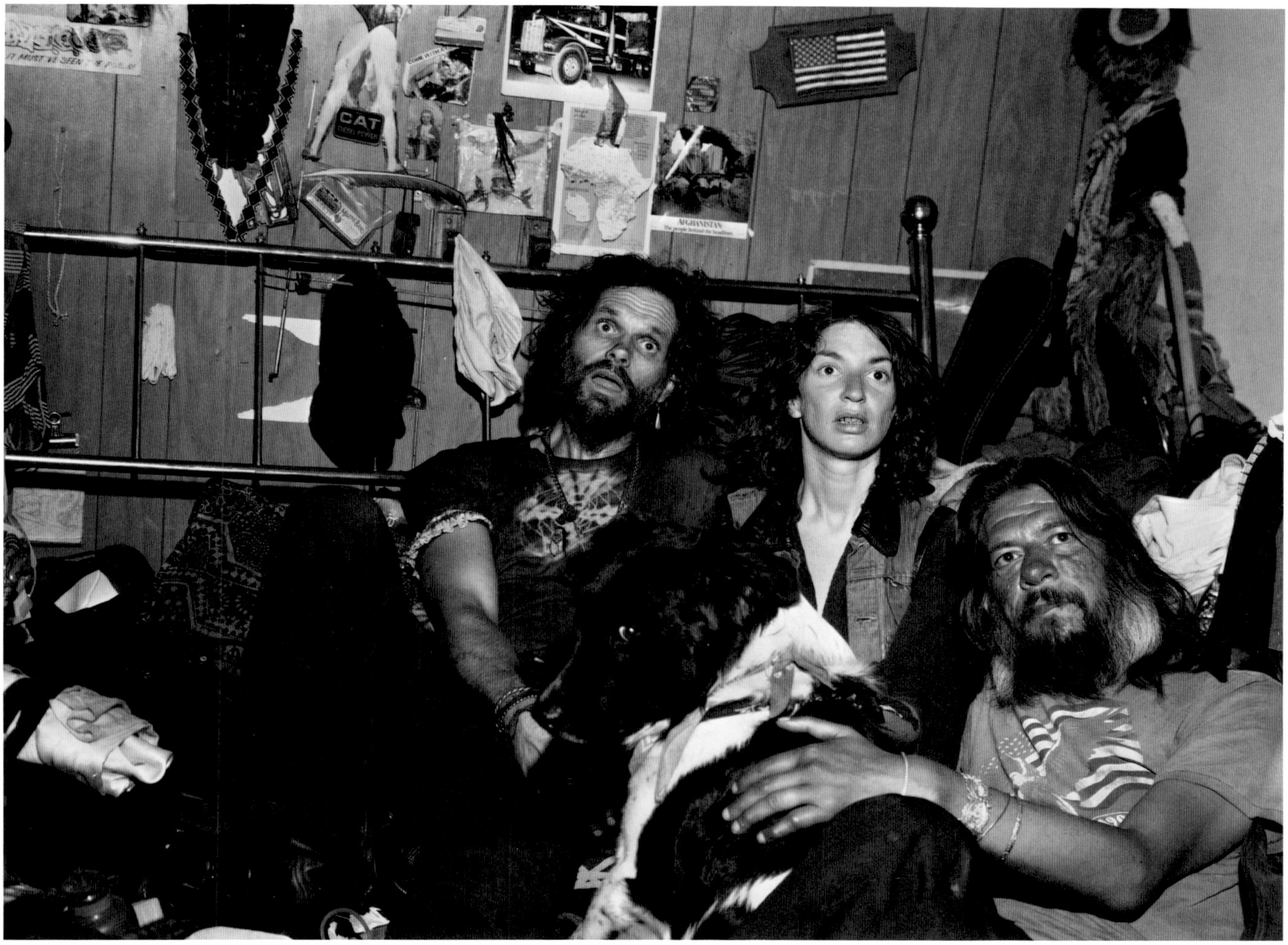
CAT

He remembered how once an old man had drunk too much and Cecily said to him baby you shouldn't have no more and the old man swore and started wobbling out the door and Cecily said can I call you a cab? and he said no I can make it on my own two fucking pins thank you and he squeezed through that heavy door like a bug emerging from an almost-closed desk drawer and he took a step outside and another and fell and smashed his head open on the sidewalk . . .

WHORES FOR GLORIA

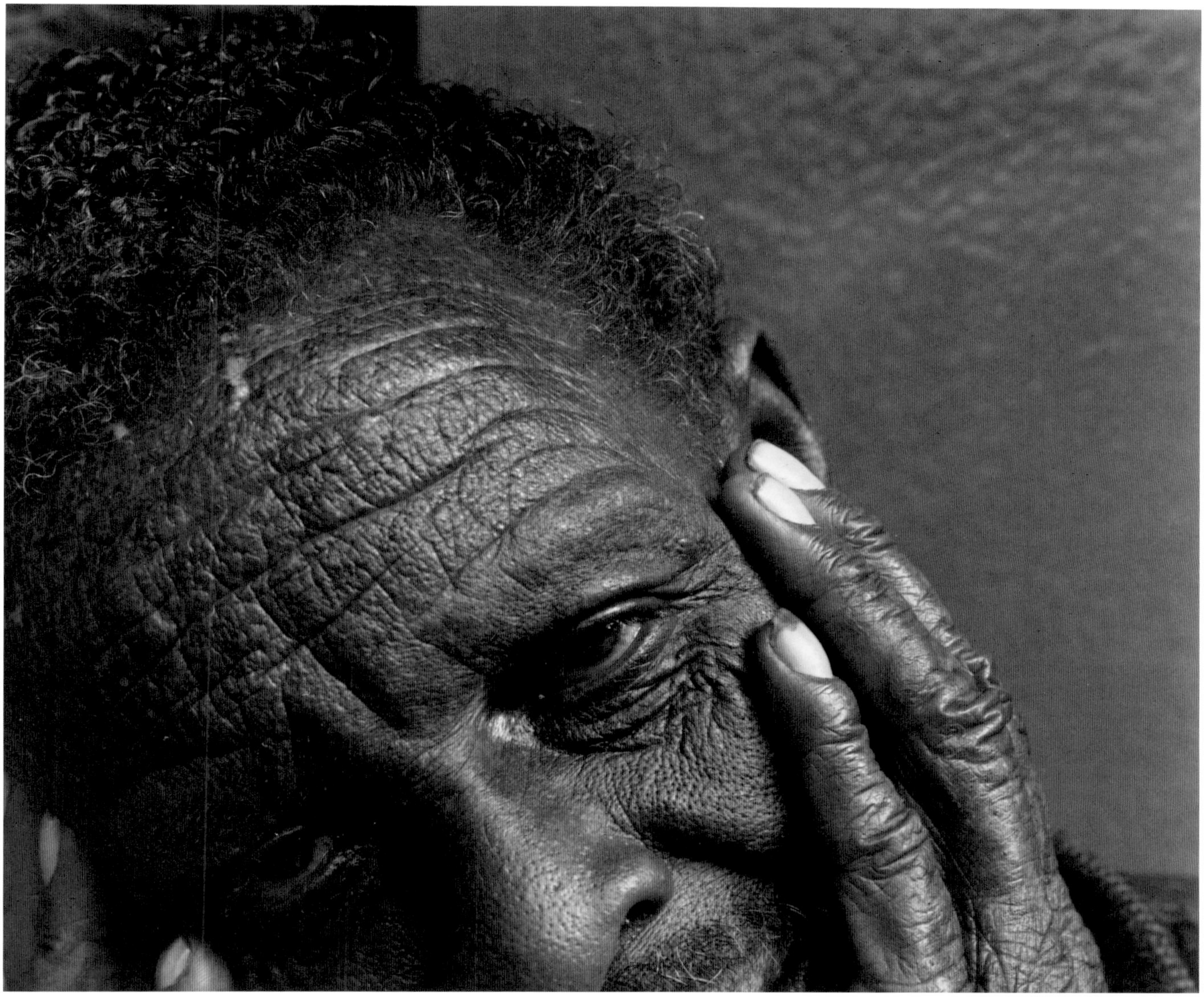

PAGE	DESCRIPTION	LOCATION	YEAR
Page 9	Lee Chain bra	San Francisco	1992
Page 11	Shizue heart chain in mouth, AKA Tokyo Girl	Tenderloin, San Francisco	1987
Page 13	Lee & Marilyn	Haight Street, San Francisco	1986
Page 15	Howard, Cosmic Commander of Wrestling	San Francisco	1992
Page 17	Cammie's Pierced Tongue	San Francisco	1992
Page 19	Love Bar	Thailand	1993
Page 21	Thai boxing: On assignment for Spin magazine	Thailand	1993
Page 23	Arsenal	San Francisco	1989
Page 25	Halloween	Haight Street, San Francisco	1986
Page 27	Bag's Face	Haight Street, San Francisco	1986
Page 29	L.A. Frank & Jim Mange Laundry Mat	Haight Street, San Francisco	1986
Page 31	Flag Day	Baker Street, San Francisco	1989
Page 33	Dickie and his Radio	Ellis Street, San Francisco	1986
Page 35	Bags & Terry Bash	Haight & Masonic, San Francisco	1985
Page 37	Skinhead Hill	Buena Vista Park	1984
Page 39	Little Dagger & Bones	San Francisco	1987
Page 41	Marisa	Haight Street, San Francisco	1985
Page 43	Marisa & surfer (surfer unknown, walked into photograph)	Ocean Beach, San Francisco	1985
Page 45	The Kiss	Haight Street, San Francisco	1985
Page 47	Marisa & Brit	San Francisco	1990
Page 49	Marisa & Curby	Haight Street, San Francisco	
Page 51	Babysitter, Drew & Christopher Jr.	San Francisco	1987
Page 53	Mary with beads	Tenderloin, San Francisco	1984
Page 55	Untitled I	Haight Street, San Francisco	1986
Page 57	Falese	Tenderloin, San Francisco	1988
Page 59	Untitled II	Tenderloin, San Francisco	1988
Page 61	Gorgeous	Tenderloin, San Francisco	1992
Page 63	Lona & Camel's head	Tenderloin, San Francisco	1992
Page 65	Miss J and Mis Gittings	San Francisco	1988
Page 67	Nick & Kim Shooting Speedball	Tenderloin, San Francisco	1988
Page 69	Japanese girl	San Francisco	1991
Page 71	Diamond on car	Tenderloin, San Francisco	1988
Page 73	Miss J.	San Francisco	1987
Page 75	Kim	Tenderloin, San Francisco	1988
Page 77	The Wrecking Crew	Golden Gate Park, San Francisco	1985
Page 79	Jimbo sleeping	Golden Gate Park, San Francisco	1986
Page 81	Market St.	San Francisco	1984
Page 83	Bill & Derick	Buena Vista Park, San Francisco	1985
Page 85	Laddie, King of the Hobos	U.S.A.	1987
Page 87	Dan Moyer, 23 years of electro shock	Haight Street, San Francisco	1984
Page 89	SSI, Linda	Haight Street, San Francisco	1984
Page 91	Judge's eyes	Oakland, California	1989
Page 93	Just after shooting speed	Haight Street, San Francisco	1987
Page 95	Edward	Haight Street, San Francisco	1984